MW00659397

Hospice/Palliative Care Training for Physicians

# Pocket Guide to Hospice/Palliative Medicine

© 2003

American Academy of Hospice and Palliative Medicine
4700 W. Lake Avenue, Glenview, IL 60025-1485

 Published in the United States by the American Academy of Hospice and Palliative Medicine, 4700 W. Lake Avenue, Glenview, IL 60025-1485.



ISBN 1-889296-35-X
Printed in the United States of America

**Cover image reproduced with permission of Deidre Scherer**

Deidre Scherer's fabric and thread images on aging have appeared in more than 100 individual and group shows including her solo exhibition at The Baltimore Museum of Art. With a Fine Arts Fellowship from the Open Society Institute, she completed her series of six life-sized panels, "Surrounded by Family and Friends." Scherer's work promotes an open dialogue about aging and dying as a natural part of life within the context of community and relationship. www.dscherer.com

Hospice/Palliative Care Training for Physicians

# Pocket Guide to Hospice/Palliative Medicine

## Authors

**Porter Storey, MD FACP FAAHPM**
Associate Professor of Medicine
Section of Geriatrics
Baylor College of Medicine

Consultant in the Department of Symptom Control and Palliative Care
University of Texas MD Anderson Cancer Center

Medical Director
Palliative Care Services
St. Luke's Episcopal Hospital
Houston, TX

**Carol F. Knight, EdM**
Knight Consultants
Austin, TX

**Ronald S. Schonwetter, MD FACP CMD FAAHPM**
Professor and Director
Division of Geriatric Medicine
Department of Internal Medicine
University of South Florida College of Medicine

Chief Medical Officer
LifePath Hospice and Palliative Care, Inc.
Tampa, FL

# Acknowledgments

The authors and the American Academy of Hospice and Palliative Medicine (AAHPM) are deeply grateful to the following reviewers for their participation in the development of this Pocket Guide. Their extensive comments and thoughtful suggestions greatly improved its contents. We also want to express special thanks to all of the practicing physicians, fellows, residents, and medical students who participated in developing and evaluating AAHPM's physician training self-study program, *Hospice/Palliative Medicine Training for Physicians: Self-Study Program*, from which the tables and figures in this Pocket Guide were taken. We also want to express special thanks to Gary S. Reiter, MD, and Carla S. Alexander, MD, co-authors of *UNIPAC Seven: The Hospice/Palliative Medicine Approach to Caring for Patients With HIV/AIDS*, and to Gerri Frager, MD, and Marcia Levetown, MD, co-authors of *UNIPAC Eight: The Hospice/Palliative Medicine Approach to Caring for Pediatric Patients*.

## Reviewers

**Robert M. Arnold, MD**
Chief, Section of Palliative Care and Medical Ethics
University of Pittsburgh Medical Center
Pittsburgh, PA

**Eduardo Bruera, MD**
Chair, Symptom Control and Palliative Medicine
MD Anderson Cancer Center
Houston, TX

**George Davis, MD**
Medical Director
Community Hospice
Albany, NY

**Laurel Herbst, MD**
Vice-President, Medical Affairs
San Diego Hospice
San Diego, CA

**David McGrew, MD**
President, Hospice and Palliative Physician Services, and
Medical Director, Hernando-Pasco Hospice, Inc.
Hudson, FL

**Paul Rousseau, MD**
Associate Chief of Staff
Geriatrics/Ext Care
Carl P. Hayden VA Medical Center
Phoenix, VA

**Sue Warren, MD**
Medical Director
Kanawha Hospice Care
Charleston, WV

**David I. Wollner, MD FACP**
Director Palliative Care Services
VA NY Harbor Health Care System
New York, NY

# AAHPM Physician Training Programs

The *Pocket Guide to Hospice/Palliative Medicine* is one component of a comprehensive physician-training program under development by the American Academy of Hospice and Palliative Medicine (AAHPM). The Academy recognizes the need for educational materials addressing hospice/palliative medicine and has designed its physician-training programs to meet its own education goals as well as those of the National Cancer Institute. Components of the training programs include:

## Hospice/Palliative Medicine Training for Physicians: Self-Study Program

The self-study program consists of a series of modules, or UNIPACs, each of which follows the recommended format for self-instructional learning, including behavioral objectives, a pretest, reading material, clinical situations for demonstrating knowledge application, a posttest, and references. The self-study program was made possible with federal funds from the National Cancer Institute's Cancer Education Grant Program, Grant # CA66771. The following UNIPACs are approved for CME credit:

- *UNIPAC One: The Hospice/Palliative Medicine Approach to End-of-Life Care*
- *UNIPAC Two: Alleviating Psychological and Spiritual Pain in the Terminally Ill*
- *UNIPAC Three: Assessment and Treatment of Pain in the Terminally Ill*
- *UNIPAC Four: Management of Selected Non-pain Symptoms in the Terminally Ill*
- *UNIPAC Five: Caring for the Terminally Ill—Communication and the Physician's Role on the Interdisciplinary Team*
- *UNIPAC Six: Ethical and Legal Decision Making When Caring for the Terminally Ill*
- *UNIPAC Seven: The Hospice/Palliative Medicine Approach to Caring for Patients with HIV/AIDS*
- *UNIPAC Eight: The Hospice/Palliative Medicine Approach to Caring for Pediatric Patients*

## *Pocket Guide to Hospice/Palliative Medicine*

The *Pocket Guide to Hospice/Palliative Medicine* is a concise, clinically oriented reference designed for residents and practicing physicians. It consists of tables and assessment tools selected primarily from the eight UNIPACs that compose the Academy's self-study program, *Hospice/Palliative Care Training for Physicians: A Self-Study Program*. Development of the Pocket Guide was made possible with federal funds from the National Cancer Institute's Cancer Education Grant Program, Grant #CA66771.

## *Hospice and Palliative Medicine: Core Curriculum and Review Syllabus*

The core curriculum and review syllabus, *Hospice and Palliative Medicine: Core Curriculum and Review Syllabus*, presents the core elements of hospice and palliative medicine identified by the Institute of Medicine as essential for effective end-of-life care. The document consists of a series of modules, each of which includes a brief narrative summary of a specific topic, objectives, and references. The curriculum is the first in the United States developed primarily by palliative medicine physicians.

## *Primer of Palliative Care*

The *Primer of Palliative Care* is a brief introduction to palliative care that covers the history of hospice, the basic elements of hospice and palliative care, pain and symptom management techniques, and alleviation of psychological, social, and spiritual distress. The primer includes an annotated bibliography.

For more information on the Academy's physician training programs, please call AAHPM at 847/375-4712, or fax 847/375-6312.

# Goals and Evaluation of the Pocket Guide

## Goals

The Pocket Guide is a concise, clinically oriented reference that describes palliative medicine interventions for improving a patient's quality of life, particularly at the end of life. The Pocket Guide is targeted to medical residents and practicing physicians not already expert in end-of-life care. It complements other, more in-depth educational materials developed by the Academy, including the self-study program, *Hospice/Palliative Medicine Training for Physicians: A Self-Study Program.* If the Pocket Guide provides clinicians with useful information and encourages them to learn more about the dynamic fields of palliative medicine and end-of-life care, it will meet its goals.

As part of its commitment to improving the care of dying patients, the American Academy of Hospice and Palliative Medicine develops educational programs to enhance physician competence in palliative medicine interventions at the end of life. One of its programs, *Hospice/Palliative Medicine Training for Physicians: A Self-Study Program*, consists of a series of CME-approved monographs, or UNIPACs, each of which addresses an aspect of hospice/palliative medicine.[1-8]

The *Self-Study Program* encourages physicians to use existing knowledge to prevent and relieve pain and other symptoms. It also encourages the use of assessment tools and the development of outcome measures, both integral to the effective practice of hospice/palliative medicine. Although the burden on patients of completing assessments must always be considered, they should be used whenever possible because they encourage careful observation, consistent assessments, effective treatment, and the development of comparative standards—all components of good care at the end of life.

## Evaluation

Please use this evaluation form to rate the Pocket Guide according to the five criteria listed below, then mail or fax the form to the Academy at the address below.

| | | | | |
|---|---|---|---|---|
| Currency of information | __Excellent | __Good | __Fair | __Poor |
| Clarity of presentation | __Excellent | __Good | __Fair | __Poor |
| Content of material | __Excellent | __Good | __Fair | __Poor |
| Effectiveness of teaching method | __Excellent | __Good | __Fair | __Poor |
| Relevance to my practice | __Excellent | __Good | __Fair | __Poor |

Suggestions for improving the enduring material:

Mail or fax to:
American Academy of Hospice and Palliative Medicine
4700 W. Lake Avenue
Glenview, IL 60025-1485
Fax: 847/734-8671

# Table of Contents

## List of Tables

## List of Figures

# 1. The Palliative Medicine Approach to End-of-Life Care

As the population of the United States ages, clinicians will be faced with rapidly growing numbers of patients with advanced illnesses. The entire healthcare system is likely to be challenged by increasing demands for optimal care voiced by patients with higher expectations for pain and symptom management, whole-person care, and inclusion in decision making.

A critical nationwide need exists for end-of-life care that offers alternatives to assisted suicide. The Institute of Medicine has made several strong recommendations, including the following:

- "People with advanced potentially fatal illnesses and those close to them should be able to expect and receive reliable, skillful, and supportive care."
- "A continuing public discussion is essential to develop a better understanding of the modern experience of dying, the options available to patients and families, and the obligations of communities to those approaching death."
- "Health professionals must commit themselves to improving care for dying patients and to using existing knowledge effectively to prevent and relieve pain and other symptoms."[9]

Hospice/palliative medicine is much more than calculating equianalgesic dosages, choosing adjuvant drugs to control specific pain syndromes, and educating patients about the likely side effects of opioid therapy. It is multidimensional and based on complex, dynamic relationships. Calculating equianalgesic doses of various opioids is easy; remaining present with the anguish of a parent whose child is dying is infinitely more difficult.

## Definitions

To establish a common ground of meaning, the *Pocket Guide* begins with definitions of several terms associated with palliative medicine (see **Table 1**, page 5).

The term *palliative care* refers to whole-person care for patients whose diseases are not responsive to curative treatment. Palliative care usually is provided by an interdisciplinary team of physicians, nurses, social workers, chaplains, and other healthcare professionals.

*Palliative treatments* include all types of measures, including very aggressive ones, to control pain and other distressing symptoms.

The term *palliative medicine* refers to a specialized area of medicine that addresses care for patients whose diseases are not responsive to curative treatment. In the United States, physicians practicing palliative medicine in hospice settings often refer to their area of expertise as *hospice/palliative medicine.*

The term *hospice* refers to a program that uses an interdisciplinary team of healthcare professionals to provide comprehensive palliative care specifically for terminally ill patients.

## Principles of Hospice Care

**Table 2**, page 6, lists Dame Cicely Saunders' principles of hospice care. Dame Saunders usually is credited with developing the art and science of modern hospice care. She pioneered the use of oral opioids to control pain and developed the concept of *total pain* to describe the all-encompassing physical, emotional, spiritual, and social distress experienced by many dying patients. Dr. Saunders also established physician training programs to improve competence in palliative medicine. She formulated the basic principles of hospice care, including the need for vigilant attention to the details of patient care and careful research to support claims about an intervention's effectiveness.

## Models of Palliative Care

The basic components of palliative care—comprehensive pain and symptom control, spiritual care, psychosocial care, grief and bereavement support, and interdisciplinary team work—are appropriate and necessary from the time of diagnosis to the time of death for all patients, particularly for children with life-limiting conditions.[16,17] Palliative interventions can improve a patient's quality of life (QOL), regardless of diagnosis or the ultimate goal of care. To care for patients effectively, physicians must provide palliative interventions appropriate for the patient's immediate situation. If and when the goal of prolonging life becomes unduly burdensome, the patient's treatment plan can be modified to further emphasize palliative interventions. **Figure 1** and **Figure 2**, page 7 describe old and new models of palliative care services. **Table 3**, page 8 describes three forms of palliative care as described in the Victoria model.

## Quality of Life

### Assessing Quality of Life

Improving a patient's QOL is the ultimate goal of palliative medicine. A one-time score on an assessment scale does not provide reliable information about a patient's quality of life; however, comparing a patient's responses over time to the same QOL assessment tool is likely to reveal important information. As patients cope with the effects of profound illness, their assessment scores are likely to diminish. Significant decreases are less likely to occur when pain and other symptoms are effectively controlled and when emotional and spiritual support is provided.

QOL assessments offer diagnostic and therapeutic benefits. In terms of diagnosis, assessments may reveal uncontrolled pain, a significant predictor of poor QOL. In terms of therapy, just the process of completing a QOL assessment tool can change a patient's perspective on issues related to living and dying, particularly as life comes to a close.

In addition to tracking an individual's QOL over time, assessment tools are useful for comparing the QOL of large populations (e.g., comparing the QOL of a large group of nursing home patients with that of a large group of patients in hospice/palliative care inpatient units). **Tables 4** and **5**, pages 9–14 are examples of QOL scales.

### Developmental Aspects of Death and Dying

**Table 6**, page 15 describes the developmental tasks associated with adequate QOL as death approaches. For more information, see *UNIPAC One: The Hospice/Palliative Medicine Approach to End-of-Life Care*[1] and *UNIPAC Eight: The Hospice/Palliative Medicine Approach to Caring for Pediatric Patients.*[8]

## The Medicare Hospice Benefit

See **Table 7**, page 16 for eligibility criteria. See **Table 8**, page 17 for a comparison of the Medicare hospice benefit and Medicare home care benefit.

## Determining Prognosis

**Tables 9–13** outline principles, performance scales, and guidelines for determining prognosis.

- **Table 9**, page 18: Determining prognosis and prognostic factors for terminally ill patients.
- **Table 10**, page 19: Karnofsky Performance Status Scale.
- **Table 11**, page 20: Eastern Cooperative Oncology group performance status scale.
- **Table 12**, page 21: Palliative Performance Scale.
- **Table 13**, pages 22–25: Summary of the National Hospice Organization's Guidelines for predicting prognosis of 6 months or less.

## Table 1. Definitions of Words Associated with Palliative Medicine

- **Palliative care** is active total care of patients whose diseases are not responsive to curative treatment. Symptom control is paramount and includes the alleviation of symptoms whether they are physical, psychological, social, or spiritual. Total palliative care usually involves an interdisciplinary team of healthcare professionals who provide coordinated medical, nursing, social work, and spiritual care services. The goal of palliative care is the achievement of the best possible quality of life for patients and their families. Many aspects of palliative care also are applicable earlier in the course of an illness in conjunction with anticancer treatment.[10]
- **Palliative care** is the comprehensive management of physical, social, spiritual, and existential needs of patients, in particular those with incurable, progressive illnesses. Palliative care affirms life and regards dying as a natural process that is a profoundly personal experience for the individual and the family. The goal of palliative care is to achieve the best possible quality of life through relief of suffering, control of symptoms, and restoration of functional capacity while remaining sensitive to personal, cultural, and religious values, beliefs, and practices.[11]
- **Palliative treatments** are treatments and interventions that enhance comfort and improve the quality of a patient's life. No specific therapy is excluded from consideration. The test of a palliative treatment lies in the agreement by the patient, physician, primary caregiver, and an interdisciplinary team of healthcare professionals that the treatment's expected outcome is relief from distressing symptoms, easing of pain, or enhancement of quality of life. The decision to intervene with an active palliative treatment is based on the treatment's ability to meet a stated goal rather than its effect on the underlying disease. The needs of each patient are continually assessed, and all treatment options are explored and evaluated within the context of the patient's values and symptoms.[12]
- **Palliative medicine** is the study and management of patients with active, progressive, far-advanced disease for whom the prognosis is limited and the focus of care is quality of life.[13] **Hospice/palliative medicine** is the study and management of patients with active, progressive, far-advanced disease for whom the prognosis is limited and the focus of care is quality of life. The discipline recognizes the multidimensional nature of suffering, responds with care that addresses all dimensions of suffering, and communicates in language that conveys mutuality, respect, and interdependence.[14]
- **Hospice programs** provide palliative care to terminally ill patients and supportive services to their families and significant others, 24 hours a day, 7 days a week, in both home- and facility-based settings. Physical, social, spiritual, and emotional care is provided during the last stages of illness, during the dying process, and during bereavement by a medically directed interdisciplinary team consisting of patients/families, professionals, and volunteers.[12]

**Table 2. Saunders' Principles of Hospice Care** [15]

- A clinical team is needed if expert control of symptoms is to be maintained.
- The hospice team involves the paramedical disciplines.
- Skilled and experienced team nursing is required.
- Methodical recording and analysis should monitor clinical practice and, with relevant research where possible, lead to soundly based practice and teaching.
- Some form of home care must be developed and fully integrated with the community services already established.
- A bereavement follow-up service should be included.
- Teaching in all aspects of terminal care should be included.
- Imaginative use of available architecture should create a supportive environment.
- An efficient and approachable administration is essential to any field of human need; it provides a sense of security to patients, families, and staff.
- Hospices should consider a mixed group of patients, including those with progressive chronic illnesses, chronic pain, and in some cases, frailty and old age.
- Readiness for the personal cost of commitment to a continuous search for meaning is essential.

## Figure 1. Old Model of Palliative Care Services

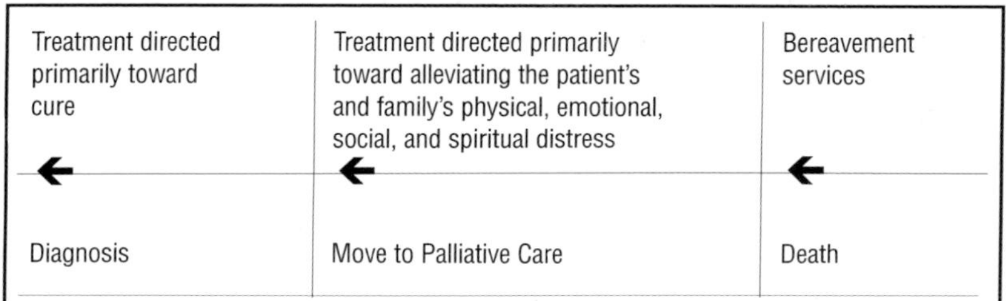


Adapted from *Palliative Care Services. Report of the Subcommittee Branch on Institutional Program Guidelines. Health Services and Promotion Branch, Health and Welfare, Canada; 1989.*[18]

## Figure 2. New Model of Palliative Care Services

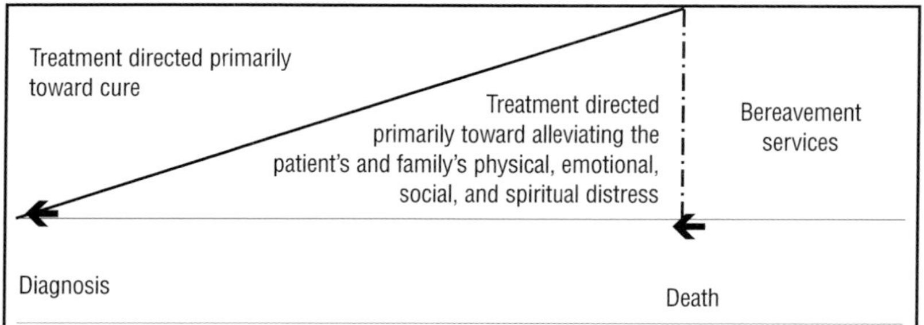


Adapted from *Palliative Care Services. Report of the Subcommittee Branch on Institutional Program Guidelines. Health Services and Promotion Branch, Health and Welfare, Canada; 1989.*[18]

## Table 3. The Victoria Model—Three Forms of Palliative Care [19]

- **Active palliation:** Active palliation includes active investigations and aggressive treatments that modify the disease. Treatments are not aimed at extending life, but extension may occur. Examples include chemotherapy, hormonal therapy, aggressive antibiotic therapy, radiation therapy, and steroids, all of which offer symptom relief but also may prolong life. Active palliative treatments can be invasive and usually require inpatient care or repeated office visits. If complications arise, they usually are treated aggressively.
- **Comfort palliation:** Most terminally ill patients live and die comfortably with comfort palliation. Interventions are noninvasive and include drug therapies and other measures to relieve symptoms instead of modifying the disease. Prolonged life is not intended but may occur due to adequate symptom relief and emotional support. Drug therapies include opioids, anxiolytics, antidepressants, nonsteroidal antiinflammatory drugs, and steroids. Other interventions include relaxation, short-term psychotherapy, grief counseling, and spiritual support that focuses on renewing the patient's sense of purpose, meaning, and hope. Most care is provided at home, although some inpatient care or respite care may be needed. Complications usually are treated with noninvasive palliative interventions.
- **Urgent palliation:** Urgent palliation is necessary when symptom emergencies occur, when patients experience moderate to severe symptoms, or when sudden complications arise. The goal of urgent palliation is to relieve symptoms as quickly as possible so the patient does not endure uncontrolled symptoms for any significant time or die with uncontrolled pain. Interventions are aggressive and often rely on subcutaneous or intravenous routes. Medications include opioids, anxiolytics, and neuroleptics. Dosages may be much higher than many physicians usually prescribe and are rapidly titrated to relieve symptoms as quickly as possible. When comfort is achieved, dosages are maintained or gradually reduced as long as comfort is maintained. When urgent palliation is used effectively, patients rarely experience a crescendo of pain toward the end of life. If uncontrolled symptoms do appear as death approaches, urgent palliation is mandatory, and sedation may be necessary to achieve relief. Urgent palliation requires experience, skill, judgment, and courage. It often requires care in an inpatient setting but may be provided in a home setting with continuous supervision and support. Relief of suffering is the intent of urgent palliative care, not shortening life.

**Table 4. McGill Quality-of-Life Questionnaire**[20]

***Over the past 2 days,***

1. One troublesome symptom is ______________.
   0 1 2 3 4 5 6 7 8 9 10
   No problem — Tremendous problem

2. Another troublesome symptom is ______________.
   0 1 2 3 4 5 6 7 8 9 10
   No problem — Tremendous problem

3. A third troublesome symptom is ______________.
   0 1 2 3 4 5 6 7 8 9 10
   No problem — Tremendous problem

4. Physically, I felt ______________.
   0 1 2 3 4 5 6 7 8 9 10
   Terrible — Well

5. I was depressed.
   0 1 2 3 4 5 6 7 8 9 10
   Not at all — Extremely

6. I was nervous or worried.
   0 1 2 3 4 5 6 7 8 9 10
   Not at all — Extremely

7. How much of the time did you feel sad?
   0 1 2 3 4 5 6 7 8 9 10
   Never — Always

8. When I think about the future, I am ______________.
   0 1 2 3 4 5 6 7 8 9 10
   Not afraid — Constantly terrified

9. My personal existence is ______________.
   0 1 2 3 4 5 6 7 8 9 10
   Utterly meaningless and without purpose — Very purposeful and meaningful

*continued*

**Table 4. McGill Quality-of-Life Questionnaire[20]** *(continued)*

***Over the past 2 days,***

10. In achieving life goals, I have ______________.

| | | |
|---|---|---|
| Made no progress whatsoever | 0 1 2 3 4 5 6 7 8 9 10 | Progressed to complete fulfillment |

11. My life to this point has been ______________.

| | | |
|---|---|---|
| Completely worthless | 0 1 2 3 4 5 6 7 8 9 10 | Very worthwhile |

12. I have ______________.

| | | |
|---|---|---|
| No control over my life | 0 1 2 3 4 5 6 7 8 9 10 | Complete control over my life |

13. I feel good about myself as a person.

| | | |
|---|---|---|
| Completely disagree | 0 1 2 3 4 5 6 7 8 9 10 | Completely agree |

14. To me, every day seems to be ______________.

| | | |
|---|---|---|
| A burden | 0 1 2 3 4 5 6 7 8 9 10 | A gift |

15. The world is ______________.

| | | |
|---|---|---|
| An impersonal, unfeeling place | 0 1 2 3 4 5 6 7 8 9 10 | Caring and responsive to my needs |

16. I feel supported.

| | | |
|---|---|---|
| Not at all | 0 1 2 3 4 5 6 7 8 9 10 | Completely |

The McGill Quality of Life Questionnaire; A measure of quality of life appropriate for people with advanced disease. A preliminary study of validity and acceptability. *Palliat Med. 1995;9(3)*:207–219. Reprinted with permission.

## Table 5. Measuring the Quality of Life of Seriously Ill Patients[21]

### Instructions to Patient

***I'd like you to think back over the last month. Please tell me the three physical symptoms or problems that have bothered you the most during that time. Some examples are pain, nausea, lack of energy, confusion, depression, anxiety, and shortness of breath.***

Symptom #1________________________ Symptom #3________________________

Symptom #2________________________

If no symptoms were elicited, then state the following: "So, just to be sure, over the last month, you have had no physical or emotional symptoms that bothered you."

If correct, skip to question #5.

**Which of these symptoms or problems has bothered you the most this past week?**

1. During the last week, how often have you experienced ________________?

| *Rarely* | *A few times* | *Fairly often* | *Very often* | *Most of the time* |
|---|---|---|---|---|
| 1 | 2 | 3 | 4 | 5 |

2. During the last week, on average, how severe has ________________ been?

| *Very mild* | *Mild* | *Moderate* | *Severe* | *Very severe* |
|---|---|---|---|---|
| 1 | 2 | 3 | 4 | 5 |

3. During the last week, how much has ________________ interfered with your ability to enjoy your life?

| *Not at all* | *A little bit* | *A moderate amount* | *Quite a bit* | *Completely* |
|---|---|---|---|---|
| 1 | 2 | 3 | 4 | 5 |

4. How worried are you about ________________ occurring in the future?

| *Not at all* | *A little bit* | *A moderate amount* | *Quite a bit* | *Completely* |
|---|---|---|---|---|
| 1 | 2 | 3 | 4 | 5 |

5. In general, how important are your physical symptoms or problems to your overall quality of life?

| *Not at all* | *A little bit* | *A moderate amount* | *Quite a bit* | *Completely* |
|---|---|---|---|---|
| 1 | 2 | 3 | 4 | 5 |

**Below is a list of statements that other people with a serious illness have said may be important. Please tell me how true each statement is for you.**

6. I have as much information as I want about my illness.

| *Not at all* | *A little bit* | *A moderate amount* | *Quite a bit* | *Completely* |
|---|---|---|---|---|
| 1 | 2 | 3 | 4 | 5 |

*continued*

## Table 5. Measuring the Quality of Life of Seriously Ill Patients[21] *(continued)*

7. Although I cannot control certain aspects of my illness, I have a sense of control about my treatment decisions.

| *Not at all* | *A little bit* | *A moderate amount* | *Quite a bit* | *Completely* |
|---|---|---|---|---|
| 1 | 2 | 3 | 4 | 5 |

8. I participate as much as I want in the decisions about my care.

| *Not at all* | *A little bit* | *A moderate amount* | *Quite a bit* | *Completely* |
|---|---|---|---|---|
| 1 | 2 | 3 | 4 | 5 |

9. Beyond my illness, my doctor has a sense of who I am as a person.

| *Not at all* | *A little bit* | *A moderate amount* | *Quite a bit* | *Completely* |
|---|---|---|---|---|
| 1 | 2 | 3 | 4 | 5 |

10. In general, I know what to expect about the course of my illness.

| *Not at all* | *A little bit* | *A moderate amount* | *Quite a bit* | *Completely* |
|---|---|---|---|---|
| 1 | 2 | 3 | 4 | 5 |

11. As my illness progresses, I know where to go to get answers to my questions.

| *Not at all* | *A little bit* | *A moderate amount* | *Quite a bit* | *Completely* |
|---|---|---|---|---|
| 1 | 2 | 3 | 4 | 5 |

12. In general, how important is feeling like an active participant in your health care to your overall quality of life?

| *Not at all* | *A little bit* | *A moderate amount* | *Quite a bit* | *Completely* |
|---|---|---|---|---|
| 1 | 2 | 3 | 4 | 5 |

13. I spend as much time as I want with my family.

| *Not at all* | *A little bit* | *A moderate amount* | *Quite a bit* | *Completely* |
|---|---|---|---|---|
| 1 | 2 | 3 | 4 | 5 |

14. There is someone in my life with whom I can share my deepest thoughts.

| *Not at all* | *A little bit* | *A moderate amount* | *Quite a bit* | *Completely* |
|---|---|---|---|---|
| 1 | 2 | 3 | 4 | 5 |

15. In general, how important are your personal relationships to your overall quality of life?

| *Not at all* | *A little bit* | *A moderate amount* | *Quite a bit* | *Completely* |
|---|---|---|---|---|
| 1 | 2 | 3 | 4 | 5 |

16. In general, how important is feeling connected to others to your overall quality of life?

| *Not at all* | *A little bit* | *A moderate amount* | *Quite a bit* | *Completely* |
|---|---|---|---|---|
| 1 | 2 | 3 | 4 | 5 |

*continued*

**Table 5. Measuring the Quality of Life of Seriously Ill Patients[21]** *(continued)*

17. Thoughts of dying frighten me.

| *Not at all* | *A little bit* | *A moderate amount* | *Quite a bit* | *Completely* |
|---|---|---|---|---|
| 1 | 2 | 3 | 4 | 5 |

18. I worry that my family is not prepared to cope with the future.

| *Not at all* | *A little bit* | *A moderate amount* | *Quite a bit* | *Completely* |
|---|---|---|---|---|
| 1 | 2 | 3 | 4 | 5 |

19. I have regrets about the way I have lived my life.

| *Not at all* | *A little bit* | *A moderate amount* | *Quite a bit* | *Completely* |
|---|---|---|---|---|
| 1 | 2 | 3 | 4 | 5 |

20. At times, I worry that I will be a burden to my family.

| *Not at all* | *A little bit* | *A moderate amount* | *Quite a bit* | *Completely* |
|---|---|---|---|---|
| 1 | 2 | 3 | 4 | 5 |

21. I worry about the financial strain caused by my illness.

| *Not at all* | *A little bit* | *A moderate amount* | *Quite a bit* | *Completely* |
|---|---|---|---|---|
| 1 | 2 | 3 | 4 | 5 |

22. In general, how important are concerns about the future to your overall quality of life?

| *Not at all* | *A little bit* | *A moderate amount* | *Quite a bit* | *Completely* |
|---|---|---|---|---|
| 1 | 2 | 3 | 4 | 5 |

23. I have been able to say important things to those close to me.

| *Not at all* | *A little bit* | *A moderate amount* | *Quite a bit* | *Completely* |
|---|---|---|---|---|
| 1 | 2 | 3 | 4 | 5 |

24. I make a positive difference in the lives of others.

| *Not at all* | *A little bit* | *A moderate amount* | *Quite a bit* | *Completely* |
|---|---|---|---|---|
| 1 | 2 | 3 | 4 | 5 |

25. I have been able to help others through time together, gifts, or wisdom.

| *Not at all* | *A little bit* | *A moderate amount* | *Quite a bit* | *Completely* |
|---|---|---|---|---|
| 1 | 2 | 3 | 4 | 5 |

26. I have been able to share important things with my family.

| *Not at all* | *A little bit* | *A moderate amount* | *Quite a bit* | *Completely* |
|---|---|---|---|---|
| 1 | 2 | 3 | 4 | 5 |

*continued*

**Table 5. Measuring the Quality of Life of Seriously Ill Patients**[21] *(continued)*

27. Despite my illness, I have a sense of meaning in my life.

| *Not at all* | *A little bit* | *A moderate amount* | *Quite a bit* | *Completely* |
|---|---|---|---|---|
| 1 | 2 | 3 | 4 | 5 |

28. I feel at peace.

| *Not at all* | *A little bit* | *A moderate amount* | *Quite a bit* | *Completely* |
|---|---|---|---|---|
| 1 | 2 | 3 | 4 | 5 |

29. In general, how important is contributing to others to your overall quality of life?

| *Not at all* | *A little bit* | *A moderate amount* | *Quite a bit* | *Completely* |
|---|---|---|---|---|
| 1 | 2 | 3 | 4 | 5 |

30. In general, how important is the feeling that your life is complete to your overall quality of life?

| *Not at all* | *A little bit* | *A moderate amount* | *Quite a bit* | *Completely* |
|---|---|---|---|---|
| 1 | 2 | 3 | 4 | 5 |

***Now, I have one last question.***

31. How would you rate your overall quality of life?

| *Very Poor* | *Poor* | *Fair* | *Good* | *Excellent* |
|---|---|---|---|---|
| 1 | 2 | 3 | 4 | 5 |

Reprinted with permission from Tulsky JA, Steinhauser KE, Bosworth HB, Clipp EC, McNeilly M, Christakis NA. A new instrument to measure quality at the end of life (QUAL-E). American Academy of Hospice and Palliative Medicine Annual Meeting; February 1, 2002: Palm Springs, CA.

**Table 6. Developmental Tasks at the End of Life[22]**

**Develop a renewed sense of personhood and meaning.**

- Find meaning(s) in life through life review and personal narrative.
- Develop a sense of worthiness, both in the past and in the current situation.
- Learn to accept love and caring from other people.

**Bring closure to personal and community relationships.**

- Say good-bye to family members and friends with expressions of regret, gratitude, appreciation, and affection.
- Ask for forgiveness from and grant forgiveness to estranged friends and family members so reconciliation can occur.
- Say good-bye to individuals involved in community relationships (employment, civic, and religious organizations) with expressions of regret, gratitude, forgiveness, and appreciation.

**Bring closure to worldly affairs.**

- Arrange for the transfer of fiscal, legal, and social responsibilities.

**Accept the finality of life, and surrender to the transcendent.**

- Express the depth of personal tragedy that dying may represent, and acknowledge the totality of personal loss.
- Withdraw from the world, and accept increased dependency.
- Develop a sense of awe, and accept the seeming chaos that can prefigure transcendence.

## Table 7. Eligibility Criteria for the Medicare Hospice Benefit

- **Patient is eligible for Medicare Part A.**

  Usually anyone who is 65 years of age or older, or is on hemodialysys or receives Medicare disability payments, is eligible.

- **Patient is terminally ill.**

  Two physicians must sign a statement certifying that the patient's medical prognosis is 6 months or less, if the disease runs its normal course. One of the physicians must be the hospice medical director or the hospice team physician; the other must be the patient's attending physician. When the hospice medical director serves as the patient's attending physician, only the signature of the medical director is required.

- **Patient chooses hospice care (informed consent).**

  The patient chooses hospice care and signs a Medicare hospice benefit election form, understanding that the goals of care are palliative rather than curative.

- **Care is provided by a Medicare-certified hospice program.**

  All care for the terminal illness is provided by a Medicare-certified hospice program

*Note:* To receive reimbursement from the Medicare Hospice Benefit or a state Medicaid Hospice Benefit, if one is available, hospice programs must certify that a Medicare/Medicaid-eligible patient is terminally ill (i.e., has a prognosis of 6 months or less, based on the physician's or medical director's judgment regarding the normal course of the individual's illness).[23]

## Table 8. Comparison of the Medicare Hospice and Medicare Home Care Benefits

| | Medicare Hospice | Medicare Home Health Care |
|---|---|---|
| Patient must be homebound. | no | yes |
| **Service Provided** | | |
| 100% coverage of medications to control pain and other symptoms related to the terminal illness (hospice programs can charge a 5% copayment) | yes | no |
| 100% coverage of durable medical equipment and medical supplies without a deductible or copayment | yes | no |
| Homemakers/home health aides | yes | yes |
| Inpatient respite care (hospice programs can charge a 5% copayment) | yes | no |
| Inpatient care with no deductible | yes | no |
| Continuous registered nurse care in the home during periods of medical crisis | yes | no |
| Counseling in the home for patient/family | yes | limited |
| Bereavement support | yes | no |
| Trained volunteers | yes | no |
| Professional management and supervision of care in all settings, including inpatient | yes | no |
| Ongoing pastoral counseling and spiritual support for patients and family | yes | no |
| Payment of consulting physician fees at 100% of Medicare allowance | yes | no |
| Physician, nurse, social worker, and counselor on-call availability 24 hours a day, 7 days a week | yes | no |

## Table 9. Determining Prognosis

### Principles of Prognosis

- No consistently accurate method of determining prognosis exists.
- Unless disease-specific criteria (see Table 13, pages 22–25) are available, functional and nutritional status are the best predictors of prognosis.
- Despite the lack of accurate methods for determining prognosis, estimates of life expectancy are very important to many patients and families.
- Physicians should provide interested patients and families with a relatively broad estimate of prognosis, with caveats that prognosis is not an exact science and the course of an illness often varies significantly from patient to patient.
- Prognosis may substantially influence patient/family behavior (e.g., completing a will, making funeral plans, saying good-bye to loved ones).
- To justify a referral to hospice/palliative care, documentation of clinical progression should include some of the following:
  –serial physical assessments
  –laboratory studies
  –radiological signs of progression
  –multiple emergency room visits
  –inpatient hospitalizations
  –results of home assessments

### Prognostic Factors for Terminally Ill Patients

- Weeks to Months
  alert
  declining clinical course
  increasing weakness, functional impairment
  impaired nutritional status
- Days to Weeks
  variable cognitive status
  increasing confusion and/or restlessness
  marked decline in clinical course
  nearly bed bound
- Hours to Days
  decreased and/or fluctuating levels of consciousness
  precipitous clinical decline
  decreased oral intake and urine output
  unable to turn over in bed
- Close to death
  periods of apnea
  rattling secretions in throat
  cool or mottled extremities

**Table 10. Karnofsky Performance Status Scale[24]**

| Definition | Percentage Score | Criteria |
|---|---|---|
| Able to carry on normal activity and work; no special care needed | 100 | Normal; no complaints; no evidence of disease |
| | 90 | Able to carry on normal activity; minor signs or symptoms of disease |
| | 80 | Normal activity with effort; some signs or symptoms of disease |
| Unable to work; able to live at home and care for most personal needs; varying amount of assistance needed | 70 | Able to care for self; unable to carry on normal activity or do active work |
| | 50 | Requires considerable assistance and frequent medical care |
| Unable to care for self; requires equivalent of institutional or hospital care; disease may be progressing rapidly | 40 | Disabled; requires special care and assistance |
| | 30 | Severely disabled; hospitalization indicated although death not imminent |
| | 20 | Very sick; hospital admission necessary; active supportive treatment necessary |
| | 10 | Moribund; fatal processes progressing rapidly |
| | 0 | Dead |

*Note:* The National Hospice Study reported that, in the absence of treatment, the Karnofsky Performance Scale (KPS) is the best predictor of a patient's length of survival. Patients with a KPS of 40 lived on average less than 50 days, while those with a KPS of 20 lived only 10–20 days.[25]

Karnofsky DA, Albelman WH, Craver LP, Burchenal JH. The Use of Nitrogen Mustards in the Palliative Treatment of Carcinoma. *Cancer*, 1948; 1:634–656. Reprinted with permission from Lippincott Williams and Wilkins.

**Table 11. Eastern Cooperative Oncology Group Performance Status Scale[26]**

| Grade | Definition |
|---|---|
| 0 | Fully active; able to carry on all predisease performance without restriction |
| 1 | Restricted in physically strenuous activity but ambulatory and able to carry out work of a light or sedentary nature (e.g., light housework, office work) |
| 2 | Ambulatory and capable of all self-care but unable to carry out any work activities; up and about more than 50% of waking hours |
| 3 | Capable of only limited self-care; confined to bed or chair more than 50% of waking hours |
| 4 | Completely disabled; cannot carry on any self-care; totally confined to bed or chair |

As published in Oken MM, Creech RH, Tormey DC, Horton J, Davis TE, McFadden ET, Carbone PP. Toxicity and response criteria of the Eastern Cooperative Oncology Group. *Am J Clin Cocol.* 1982; 5, 649–655. Please refer to www.ecog.org/general/perf_stat.html

**Table 12. Palliative Performance Scale (PPS)[27]**

| Percentage Score | Ambulation | Activity and Evidence of Disease | Self-Care | Nutritional Intake | Consciousness |
|---|---|---|---|---|---|
| 100 | Full | Normal activity; no evidence of disease | Full | Normal | Full |
| 90 | Full | Normal activity; some evidence of disease | Full | Normal | Full |
| 80 | Full | Normal activity with effort; significant disease | Full | Normal or reduced | Full |
| 70 | Reduced | Unable to do normal job/work; some evidence of disease | Full | Normal or reduced | Full |
| 60 | Reduced | Unable to do hobby/housework; significant disease | Occasional assistance necessary | Normal or reduced | Full or confusion |
| 50 | Mainly sit or lie | Unable to do any work; extensive disease | Considerable assistance required | Normal or reduced | Full or confusion |
| 40 | Mainly in bed | Unable to do most activities | Mainly assistance | Normal or reduced | Full or drowsy +/- confusion |
| 30 | Totally bed bound | As above | Total care | Reduced | Full or drowsy +/- confusion |
| 20 | As above | As above | Total care | Minimal sips | As above |
| 10 | As above | As above | Total care | Mouth care only | Drowsy or coma +/- confusion |
| 0 | Death | — | — | — | — |

Anderson F, Downing GM, Hill J, Casorsc L, Lerch N. Palliative Performance Scale (PPS): A new tool. *J Palliat Care.* 1996;12(1):5–11. Reprinted with permission from the *Journal of Palliative Care.* Revised to reflect version 2, www.victoriahospice.com.

## Table 13. Summary of the National Hospice Organization's Guidelines for Determining Prognosis of 6 Months or Less[28*]

| Disease | Primary Factors | Secondary Factors |
|---|---|---|
| Heart Disease | • Symptoms of recurrent heart failure or angina at rest, discomfort with any activity (NYHA Class IV)<br>• Patient already optimally treated with diuretics and vasodilators (e.g., angiotensin-converting enzyme inhibitors) | • Ejection fraction ≤ 20%<br>• Symptomatic arrhythmias<br>• History of cardiac arrest and CPR<br>• Unexplained syncope<br>• Embolic cerebrovascular accident of cardiac origin<br>• HIV disease |
| Pulmonary Disease | • Disabling dyspnea at rest<br>• Progressive pulmonary disease (e.g., increasing emergency room visits or hospitalizations for pulmonary infections and/or respiratory failure)<br>• Hypoxemia at rest on supplemental $O_2$<br>–$pO_2 \leq 55$ mm Hg on supplemental $O_2$<br>–$O_2$ sat ≤ 88% on supplemental $O_2$<br>OR<br>Hypercapnia<br>–$pCO_2 \geq 50$ mm Hg | • $FEV_1$ after bronchodilator < 30% of predicted for normal patients<br>• Decreased $FEV_1$ on serial testing > 40 ml per year<br>• Unintentional weight loss >10% of body weight in 6 months<br>• Resting tachycardia >100 beats/min in patient with severe chronic obstructive pulmonary disease<br>• Documented cor pulmonale or right heart failure due to advanced pulmonary disease |
| Dementia | • Severity of dementia ≥ FAST Stage 7-C[29]<br>–unable to walk, dress, or bathe without assistance<br>–urinary and fecal incontinence<br>–unable to speak more than six different intelligible words per day<br>• Severe comorbid condition within past 6 months<br>–aspiration pneumonia<br>–pyelonephritis<br>–septicemia<br>–multiple, progressive stage 3–4 decubiti<br>–fever after antibiotics | |

*continued*

**Table 13. Summary of the National Hospice Organization's Guidelines for Determining Prognosis of 6 Months or Less[28]*** *(continued)*

| Disease | Primary Factors | Secondary Factors |
|---|---|---|
| Dementia *(continued)* | • Unable to maintain fluid/caloric intake to sustain life<br>• If feeding tube in place, weight loss >10% in 6 months or serum albumin < 2.5 gm/dl | |
| HIV Disease (*Developed prior to highly active antiretroviral therapies. See* UNIPAC Seven.) | • CD4+ < 25 cells/µL<br>OR<br>Viral load ≥ 100,000 copies/ml<br>• Karnofsky ≤ 50%<br>• One of the following:<br>–central nervous system lymphoma<br>–progressive multifocal leukoencephalopathy<br>–advanced dementia<br>–cryptosporidiosis<br>–wasting > 33% of body weight<br>–toxoplasmosis<br>–visceral Kaposi's sarcoma, no Rx<br>–Mycobacterium avium complex, no Rx<br>–renal failure, no dialysis | • Foregoing antiretroviral and prophylatic drug Rx<br>• Chronic, persistent diarrhea for 1 year<br>• Albumin < 2.5gm/dL<br>• Age > 50 years<br>• CHF, NYHA Class IV<br>• Active substance abuse<br>Note: A Karnofsky performance score ≤ 50% indicates the patient requires considerable assistance and frequent medical care. |
| Liver Disease | • End-stage cirrhosis; not a candidate for liver transplant<br>• Prothrombin time > 5 sec over control or INR > 1.5 AND serum albumin < 2.5 g/dL<br>• At least one of the following:<br>–ascites despite diuretics and low sodium diet<br>–spontaneous bacterial peritonitis<br>–hepatorenal syndrome<br>–hepatic encephalopathy despite treatment<br>–recurrent variceal bleed | • Progressive malnutrition<br>• Muscle wasting<br>• Continued alcoholism<br>• Primary liver cancer<br>• Positive HBsAg |
| Renal Disease | • Chronic renal failure; coming off or not a candidate for dialysis<br>• Creatinine clearance < 10 cc/min (for diabetics < 15 cc/min) AND serum creatinine > 8.0 mg/dL (for diabetics > 6.0 mg/dL) | • Mechanical ventilation<br>• Malignancy—other organ system<br>• Chronic lung disease<br>• Advanced cardiac or liver disease<br>• Sepsis |

*continued*

**Table 13. Summary of the National Hospice Organization's Guidelines for Determining Prognosis of 6 Months or Less[28]* *(continued)***

| Disease | Primary Factors | Secondary Factors |
|---|---|---|
| Renal Disease *(continued)* | –Signs and symptoms associated with renal failure<br>–uremia: nausea, pruritus, confusion, or restlessness<br>–oliguria: output <400 cc/24 hours<br>–intractable hyperkalemia: serum K > 7.0<br>–uremic pericarditis<br>–hepatorenal syndrome<br>–intractable fluid overload | • Immunosuppression/ HIV disease<br>• Cachexia or albumin ≤ 3.5 gm/dL<br>• Age > 75 years<br>• Platelets < 25,000<br>• Gastrointestinal bleed<br>• Disseminated intravascular coagulation |
| Stroke and Coma | *Acute phase following cerebrovascular accident*<br>• Coma or persistent vegetative state > 3 days<br>• Any one of the following on day 3 of coma:<br>–abnormal brain stem response<br>–absent verbal response<br>–absent withdrawal to pain<br>–serum creatine >1.5 mg/dL<br>• Inability to maintain fluid/caloric intake to sustain life<br><br>*Chronic phase of cerebrovascular accident*<br>• Any one of the following:<br>–age > 70 years<br>–poststroke dementia: FAST score > 7 (unable to toilet, dress, or bathe without assistance; unable to speak more than six different intelligible words per day; and occasional urinary or fecal incontinence)<br>–Karnofsky ≤ 50%<br>–poor nutritional status | • Aspiration pneumonia<br>• Upper urinary tract infection (e.g., pyelonephritis)<br>• Sepsis<br>• Progressive, refractory stage 3–4 decubiti<br>• Fever after antibiotics<br><br>Note: A Karnofsky score ≤ 50% indicates the patient requires considerable assistance and frequent medical care. |

*continued*

**Table 13. Summary of the National Hospice Organization's Guidelines for Determining Prognosis of 6 Months or Less[28*]** *(continued)*

| Disease | Primary Factors | Secondary Factors |
|---|---|---|
| Amyotrophic Lateral Sclerosis | • Critically impaired ventilatory capacity indicated by<br>–vital capacity < 30% of predicted for normal patients<br>–significant dyspnea at rest<br>–requires $O_2$ at rest<br>–declines intubation, tracheostomy, mechanical ventilation<br>OR<br>• Rapid progression and critical nutritional impairment indicated by<br>–oral intake of nutrients/fluids insufficient to sustain life<br>–continued weight loss<br>–dehydration or hypovolemia<br>OR<br>• Rapid progression and life-threatening complications such as<br>–aspiration pneumonia<br>–upper urinary infection (i.e., pyelonephritis)<br>–sepsis<br>–multiple, progressive stage 3–4 decubiti<br>–fever recurrent after antibiotics | |

*A life-limiting condition with evidence of either disease progression and/or impaired nutritional status indicated by involuntary weight loss ≥10% of body weight in past 6 months. Serum albumin ≤ 2.5 is a helpful but not necessary factor. The goal of treatment is relief of symptoms, not cure.

# 2. Alleviation of Psychological and Spiritual Pain

## Psychological and Spiritual Pain Assessment

**Table 14**, page 29, provides general guidelines for the assessment of psychological and spiritual pain.

## Psychological Pain

### Loss and Grief

**Table 15**, page 30, lists possible losses associated with terminal illness; **Table 16**, pages 31–32, common reactions to loss; **Table 17**, page 33, the tasks of grief; **Table 18**, pages 34–35, the risk factors for complicated grief; and **Table 19**, pages 36–37, the four types of complicated grief.

### Anxiety

See **Table 20**, pages 38–39, for the symptoms, causes, and treatment of anxiety.

### Depression

Depression is common among terminally ill patients and their family caregivers.[40–42] Most cases of depression are undetected by physicians and other skilled healthcare providers, unless they systematically use a screening instrument for depression.[43,44]

The Center for Epidemiological Studies–Depression (CES-D), a widely used and validated screening tool, detects depression in patients and caregivers and can be used to monitor mood changes over time. The 10-item version of the CES-D (the Boston short form; see **Table 21**, page 40) is the briefest and simplest version.[45–47] The instrument should not be used by itself to diagnose depression. Additional questions must be asked to diagnose specific depressive disorders and plan treatment. Repeated administration of the instrument over time provides valuable information for both clinical purposes and program development. For more information, see *UNIPAC Two: Alleviating Psychological and Spiritual Pain in the Terminally Ill.*[2]

**Table 22**, pages 41–42, lists the causes, symptoms, and treatments of depression. **Table 23**, pages 43–44, describes some pharmacological agents used for treating major depression in patients with advanced disease. **Table 24**, page 45, lists risk factors for suicide in patients with advanced disease.

## Spiritual Pain

Regardless of their religious affiliation or lack thereof, people confront universal spiritual issues whenever they try to make sense of existence, suffering, and death. Spiritual pain generally occurs during times of crisis. Often it involves searching for answers to spiritual questions such as those in **Table 25**, page 46.

### Definitions of Spirituality and Religion

**Table 26**, page 46, gives possible definitions of the terms spirituality and religion. See **Table 27**, pages 47–49, for principles of spiritual assessment.

### A Spiritual Assessment Tool

**Table 28**, page 50, is an example of a spiritual assessment tool.

### Alleviation of Spiritual Pain

The basic goal of intervention is to help people access their inner spiritual resources and strengthen them. Doing so can improve their quality of life as they cope with the challenges of a terminal illness. Involving the patient's minister, rabbi, pastor, spiritual advisor, or hospice chaplain (with the patient's permission) can be very helpful. It may be essential if the patient is experiencing deep spiritual pain that requires intensive interventions from trained professionals.

Spiritual healing often involves an experience of transcendence. Kellehear (see **Table 29**, page 51) proposes three dimensions of transcendence, along with desires commonly experienced by patients as they cope with each dimension.[53] Hay (see **Table 30**, pages 52–53) describes four dimensions of spiritual pain and proposes interventions to relieve the spiritual distress associated with each dimension.[54]

## Maintaining Hope

See **Table 31**, page 54, for the Herth Hope Index. **Table 32**, pages 55–56, outlines ways in which hope can be fostered in patients, their families, and the medical staff.

## Table 14. Psychological and Spiritual Pain: General Assessment Guidelines

**Suspect psychological and spiritual pain.**

- Grief and spiritual concerns affect nearly all dying patients. The index of suspicion for the presence of psychological or spiritual pain should be high, and it should increase if the following occur:[30]
  - The patient's physical symptoms are unexplainable and do not respond to usually effective interventions.
  - The patient's emotional responses seem out of proportion to the loss.
  - Compliance with treatments is erratic.

**Establish a conducive atmosphere.**

- A comfortable and unhurried atmosphere should be established. It is important to sit down and take time to make the patient feel comfortable. A partially clothed patient sitting on a hard examination table in a cold room is unlikely to voice spiritual concerns, and few deeply troubling thoughts will be shared with a physician who remains standing by the door.
- Physicians with little experience, training, or interest in nonphysical sources of pain may send nonverbal messages conveying their discomfort or lack of interest. Patients are then unlikely to voice psychological or spiritual concerns.

**Express interest and ask specific questions.**

- Patients tend to report what they believe the physician and other members of the team are interested in hearing. Asking specific questions about psychological and spiritual concerns indicates the physician's interest and validates the importance of such concerns. When clinicians ask only about physical pain, that is what patients will report despite the presence of profound psychological or spiritual distress.[30]

**Listen for broader meanings.**

- Focusing only on physical symptoms devalues spiritual, psychological, and social pain; can reinforce a sense of distance between the patient and the practitioner; and prohibits an awareness of larger meanings. Although deconstructing an illness (i.e., separating it into discreet, smaller parts) may be appropriate in some situations, it is not appropriate when one is assessing for total pain.
- Assessments should include specific questions designed to elicit a patient's feelings and thoughts about the broader meanings of the illness and the illness's effect on the patient's entire life.[31]

## Table 15. Possible Losses Associated with Terminal Illness[32,33]

**Physical and intellectual losses**
- Short-term memory
- Mental, physical, and sexual functioning
- Limbs, other body parts, the entire body
- Sense of good health and physical well-being
- Control over personal environment and body functions

**Social losses**
- Family members
- Friends
- Political and civic life
- Religious community

**Emotional and psychological losses**
- Perceived future, hopes, and dreams
- Self-image
- Secret life
- Emotional self-control
- Privacy and freedom
- Life roles (e.g., parent, child, nurturer, chauffeur, breadwinner, cook, lover)

**Spiritual losses**
- Trust in God
- Sense of grounding or connection with the transcendent
- Sense of wholeness
- Sense of purpose, value, worth
- Sense of hope and meaning

## Table 16. Common Reactions to Loss[34–36]

**Physical**

- Tightness in chest or throat
- Hollowness in the stomach
- Oversensitivity to noise
- Dry mouth
- Breathlessness, feeling of shortness of breath
- Weakness in the muscles
- Lack of energy
- Sense of depersonalization and disconnection

**Cognitive**

- Disbelief
- Confusion and difficulty in concentrating
- Preoccupation with the deceased and obsessive thoughts related to the death
- Sense of the deceased's presence
- Brief visual and auditory hallucinations of the deceased
- Transient thoughts of not wanting to go on living or of not being able to make it through life without the deceased
- Dreams about the deceased
- Denial of the death and associated feelings of grief

**Behavioral**

- Absent-mindedness
- Social withdrawal
- Sleep disturbance
- Restless overactivity
- Crying
- Appetite disturbance
- Sighing
- Avoiding reminders of the deceased
- Visiting places and carrying objects that remind the survivor of the deceased
- Searching and calling out for the deceased
- Dreaming about the deceased
- Treasuring objects that belonged to the deceased
- High levels of fatigue with listlessness and apathy
- Disorganization

*continued*

**Table 16. Common Reactions to Loss[34–36]** *(continued)*

**Emotional**

- Sadness, frequently accompanied by tears
- Shock and numbness
- Anger at the deceased for dying, at God for allowing the death, at physicians
- Guilt and self-reproach
- Anxiety and depression
- Rapid mood changes and irritability
- Loneliness and a sense of helplessness
- Despair, anguish, and yearning for the deceased
- Disconnection from self and others, isolation, and sense of being lost
- Disconnection from the transcendent realm, spiritual disorganization, loss of faith or religious beliefs
- Sense of the world as unreasonable, unpredictable, and dangerous
- Sense of being broken, split apart, and disconnected
- Loss of purpose and direction
- Loss of hope, trust, and meaning
- Periodic thoughts of not wanting to go on living
- Relief and emancipation

**Table 17. Tasks of Grief**[35]

| |
|---|
| **Accept the reality of the loss.**<br>Accepting the reality of the loss refers to working through a normal tendency to deny that a loss has occurred. It does not imply that the bereaved person is coming to terms with the loss but refers only to an intellectual and emotional acknowledgment that a loss has actually occurred (i.e., it is not a nightmare that will end in the morning).<br>Sorting out reality is a painful but essential process that occurs before readjustment and "moving on" can begin. Clinicians can help patients and families begin to accept the reality of their loss and gain a sense of control over it by encouraging the bereaved to name all of the losses they have experienced as a result of illness or death.[37] |
| **Experience the pain of the loss.**<br>Experiencing the pain of loss means giving up attempts to deny or minimize grief and feeling the emotional reactions that accompany grieving. Because such feelings are painful, the temptation is to cut short the pain of grief—to get it over with and go on with life prematurely. Caught in their own feelings of helplessness, physicians, family members, and friends may encourage mourners to circumvent the process with medication or distraction. To recover, however, mourners need to experience the painful feelings of loss. Such feelings make the loss real; they define what was and is no more. |
| **Adjust to an environment without the deceased.**<br>Adjusting to a new environment means learning how to live without the deceased, which can be a disturbing and painful process that often takes longer than expected. As the bereaved person begins to appreciate all the roles the deceased filled (e.g., friend, confidant, lover, bill payer, bed warmer, car washer, cook), the sense of loss can be overwhelming. The bereaved may resent having to learn new tasks (e.g., grocery shopping, managing a bank account, arranging social occasions). However, with time, most people are proud of their growing independence and newly learned skills. Moving from a state of helplessness to one of responsibility for learning new skills is the basic requirement of this task. |
| **Emotionally relocate the deceased and move on with life.**<br>Emotionally relocating the deceased means that mourners begin to redirect their emotional energy from the person who died to those who are living and to satisfying hobbies and other activities. Successful relocation is associated with a gradual reorganization of life to changed circumstances. Because mourners sometimes think that recovery means forgetting the deceased, they may struggle to keep the deceased present by putting their own lives on hold. However, recovery does not mean forgetting; it means gradually adjusting the relationship with the deceased from one of presence to one of memory. |

## Table 18. Risk Factors for Complicated Grief[35,36]

**What the loss was, and who the deceased person was**

Reactions to loss vary depending on the particular meaning of the loss for a specific person. Because a terminal illness often means the approaching loss of everything a dying patient has ever known and cared about, reactions can be severe.

The loss of a spouse generally leads to protracted disorganization, while the loss of a child may evoke the most lasting and intense yearning and anger. The age of the deceased affects the bereaved's reactions to loss; the death of a child generally is associated with complicated grief for the survivors.

**The nature of the attachment**

Clinging or ambivalent relationships are associated with complicated grief, particularly when initial feelings of relief are followed by feelings of anger and guilt. Difficult grief reactions may occur when the deceased was the survivor's primary source of self-worth and self-esteem (e.g., when a dependent partner dies, the survivor may have difficulty finding a role to replace the lost role of caretaker).

**Mode of loss/death**

Losses, including deaths, that are sudden, unexpected, untimely, or multiple are more likely to result in complicated grief. Deaths associated with suicide, mutilation, or perceived threats to the survivor's life typically result in patterns of grieving characterized by attempts to avoid, repress, or delay grief for months or years at a time. The numbness and blunting that are part of the normal process of grieving may persist for much longer periods of time. Attempts to delay grief will not prevent the bereaved from experiencing high levels of ongoing anger and tension.

**Historical antecedents**

- Previous patterns of coping may be predictive of responses to a loss. However, successful integration of an expected and timely loss may not be an accurate predictor of reactions to a more traumatic loss.
- A history of psychiatric illness, including major depression or anxiety disorders, increases the risk of a difficult grieving process. Past or current threats of suicide are associated with complicated grief.
- Multiple losses can result in chronic serial grief, a devastating condition that results from the loss of several significant relationships, one soon after another.

**Personality variables**

Past or current misuse of or lack of trust in self and others.

*continued*

## Table 18. Risk Factors for Complicated Grief[35,36] *(continued)*

**Social factors**

- Frequent moves, estrangement, geographic separation from other family members, or lack of supportive networks (e.g., church or social groups) can adversely affect the grieving process. The presence of caring family members who provide support for those most affected by the loss often is a predictor of good outcome.
- A lack of cultural norms with established models for mourning can adversely affect the grieving process.

**Concurrent stresses**

Losses that result in major life changes (e.g., serious economic reversals, moves, job changes, abrupt changes in caregiving responsibilities for young children) often affect the grieving process adversely.

## Table 19. Four Types of Complicated Grief [35,38]

**Chronic grief**

Chronic grief may indicate the mourner is stuck—the process of grieving has halted.

- Grief is static (i.e., the levels of depression, anger, or guilt remain unchanged for months or years).
- The mourner has a long history of unexplained pain, depression, or anxiety that began with the loss of a loved one.

**Delayed grief**

A mourner may attempt to delay grief when losses have overwhelmed the ability to cope. Delayed grief is most common when a death is completely unexpected, particularly violent, or the result of suicide or a criminal act.

- Expressions of grief are suppressed or inhibited.
- Minor events trigger intense reactions, even years after the death.
- Responses to a recent death seem out of proportion to the degree of loss.
- Mourners are unable to talk about the deceased without fresh expressions of grief, even many years after the death.

**Masked grief**

Masked grief is likely to be present when the mourner develops the following symptoms and is unable to recognize them as related to grief:

- Avoidance of any emotion when discussing the deceased or the mourner's current situation
- Unexplained anxiety or depression
- Aberrant or maladaptive behaviors (e.g., an inability to leave the house or panic attacks)
- Disabling, nonaffective physical symptoms similar to those experienced by the deceased (e.g., pain, nausea, numbness, anorexia)
- Chronic changes in lifestyle following a death (e.g., withdrawal from friends)
- Avoidance of the grave site, nonparticipation in death-related rituals such as funerals, unwillingness to read cards of condolence, chronic unwillingness to move any of the deceased's material possessions
- Self-destructive behaviors (e.g., failure to provide for basic survival needs such as safety and nutrition, abuse of alcohol or prescription drugs)

*continued*

## Table 19. Four Types of Complicated Grief[35,38] *(continued)*

| |
|---|
| **Exaggerated grief**<br>In exaggerated grief, the mourner understands that the symptoms are related to grief but feels completely overwhelmed for long periods of time by feelings such as the following:<br>• Depression or anxiety<br>• Severe inability to concentrate<br>• Helplessness and hopelessness<br>• Worthlessness and emptiness<br>• Irrational despair<br>• Panic attacks<br>• Phobias about illness or death<br>• Mania<br>• Persistent thoughts of suicide or formation of a plan to commit suicide |

## Table 20. Anxiety: Symptoms, Causes, and Treatments[39]

| Symptoms | Causes | Treatments |
|---|---|---|
| • Persistent tenseness<br>• Inability to relax<br>• Worry, fearfulness, dread<br>• More-than-normal mood variation<br>• Poor concentration<br>• Impaired ability to assimilate or recall information<br>• Rumination, intrusive thoughts<br>• Indecisiveness<br>• Insomnia<br>• Irritability, restlessness<br>• Inability to distract self and or be distracted<br>• Panic attacks<br>• Sweating, tremor<br>• Nausea, anorexia<br>• Shortness of breath, hyperventilation | *Situational*<br>• Worry about family, finances<br>• Fear of the unknown, hospital, treatment<br>• Isolation, inadequate support<br>• Role loss, sense of uselessness<br>• Uncertainty, lack of information, misinformation<br><br>*Drug-related*<br>• Corticosteroids<br>• Drug-induced hallucinations<br>• Benzodiazepines or opioids<br>• Withdrawal states precipitated by abrupt discontinuation of benzodiazepines, alcohol, opioids<br><br>*Organic*<br>• Uncontrolled pain and other symptoms<br>• Dyspnea, hypoxia, increasing respiratory effort<br>• Weakness<br>• Hypoglycemia, sepsis, fever, hypotension<br>• Insomnia<br>• Brain tumor<br>• Adverse drug reactions such as akathisia or myoclonus | **Nonpharmacological**<br>• Multidisciplinary assessment<br>• Treatment of reversible causes<br>• Short-term psychotherapy<br>*If the above are ineffective, use medications such as the following.*<br><br>**Pharmacological**<br>**For simple anxiety:**<br>**Benzodiazepines**<br>• Diazepam 2–20 mg PO qd, bid, or tid. Peaks in 15–45 minutes. Liquid formulation available. Other routes: SL/PR/IV. Long half-life; steady plasma concentration.<br>• Lorazepam (Ativan) 0.5–2 mg PO or SL bid, tid, or qid. Peaks in 1–6 hours. Liquid available. Other routes: SL/PR/ IV. Medium half-life.<br>• Alprazolam (Xanax) 0.25–2 mg PO tid or qid. Peaks in 30 minutes. Other routes: SL/PR Short half-life.<br>• Clonazepam (Klonopin) 0.25–0.5 PO bid–tid up to 4 mg/day. Long acting. |

*continued*

**Table 20. Anxiety: Symptoms, Causes, and Treatments**[39] *(continued)*

| Symptoms | Causes | Treatments |
|---|---|---|
| | *Psychological*<br>• Denial, anger, guilt, fear<br>• Preexisting anxiety disorders (exaggerated reaction)<br>• Preexisting anxiety disorders (panic disorders, obsessive-compulsive disorder, phobias)<br>• Depression<br>• Delirium<br><br>*Causes related to patient's inner world*<br>• Existential distress, hopelessness, meaninglessness<br>• Fear of mental impairment<br>• Fear of loss of independence<br>• Fear of pain<br>• Thoughts about death<br>• Thoughts about the past (wasted opportunities, guilt) | **For anxiety with paranoia, hallucinations, or severe anxiety: Major tranquilizers**<br>• Haloperidol (Haldol) 0.5–4 mg bid and q 4 hours prn. Peaks in 3–6 hours. Liquid available. Other routes: SL/PR/SC/IV. Neuroleptic; antiemetic benefit.<br>**If the above are ineffective, or if the patient is unable to take oral medications**<br>• Midazolam (Versed) 1 mg SC/IV stat (0.5–2 mg q 2–4 hours SC). Peaks in ½–1 hour (IM). Other routes: PO/IV. Very short half-life; no drug accumulation.<br>• Opioids: add or increase dose by 50%<br>• Phenobarbital 130 mg SC daily to q 4 hours |

## Table 21. Center for Epidemiologic Studies-Depression (CES-D) Boston Short Form [45]

**Ask: Did you experience the following much of the time during the past week?**

| Yes | No | Item |
|---|---|---|
| X | | I felt depressed. |
| X | | I felt that everything I did was an effort. |
| X | | My sleep was restless. |
| | X | I was happy. |
| X | | I felt lonely. |
| X | | People were unfriendly. |
| | X | I enjoyed life. |
| X | | I felt sad. |
| X | | I felt that people disliked me. |
| X | | I could not get going. |

**Scoring:** The user sums the scores of all items. The items marked "no" are scored in reverse. A score ≥ 4 indicates a high probability of depression. A score < 3 indicates a low probability of depression.

Irwin M, Artin KH, Oxmnan MN. Screening for depression in the older adult: criterion validity of the 10-item Center for Epidemiological Studies Depression Scale. *Arch Intern Med.* 1999;159:1701–1704. ©1999, American Medical Association. Reprinted with permission.

**Table 22. Depression: Symptoms, Causes, Treatments**

| Symptoms | Causes | Treatments |
|---|---|---|
| *Psychological*<br>• Profound feelings of worthlessness<br>• Profound feelings of guilt<br>• Profound anhedonia<br>• Profound thoughts of wishing for death<br>• Profound feelings of hopelessness<br>• Suicidal ideation<br><br>*Somatic*<br>Somatic signs and symptoms are of little value in diagnosing depression in terminally ill patients, because the illness itself can produce symptoms of fatigue, loss of energy, anorexia, insomnia, and other symptoms. | *Psychiatric*<br>• Major depression<br>• Adjustment disorders<br><br>*Medical*<br>• Poorly controlled pain or other physical symptoms<br>• Drugs (e.g., opioids, corticosteroids, diazepam)<br>• Tumor involvement of central nervous system<br>• Infections (e.g., Epstein-Barr virus)<br>• Metabolic disturbances (e.g., abnormal levels of sodium or calcium)<br>• Nutritional problems (e.g., anemia, deficiencies in vitamin B12 or folate) | ***Nonpharmacological***<br>• Multidisciplinary assessments<br>• Treatment of reversible causes<br>• Short-term psychotherapy<br>*If the above are ineffective, consider medications such as the following.*<br><br>***Pharmacological***<br>**Serotonin reuptake inhibitors (SSRIs)**<br>• Less sedating and fewer autonomic side effects<br>• Temporary nausea and anxiety fairly common<br>• Less helpful in treating neuropathic pain<br>• Often reduces libido<br>• More sedating SSRIs: sertraline, paroxetine<br>• More energizing SSRIs: fluoxetine and fluvoxamine<br><br>**Tricyclic Antidepressants**<br>• Greater anticholinergic effect<br>• Neuropathic pain alleviation<br>• Low starting doses, increase slowly<br>• Therapeutic response at lower-than-usual doses in patients with advanced disease<br>• Anxiety or insomnia present: use sedating antidepressants (e.g., amitriptyline, doxepin)<br>• Psychomotor retardation present: use less sedating drugs (e.g., desipramine) |

*continued*

**Table 22. Depression: Symptoms, Causes, Treatments** *(continued)*

| Symptoms | Causes | Treatments |
|---|---|---|
| | • Endocrine disorders (e.g., hypothyroidism, adrenal insufficiency)<br>• Neurological disorders (e.g., Parkinson's disease)<br><br>*Psychological, social, spiritual*<br>• Grief<br>• Existential distress<br>• Concern about family distress<br>• Overwhelming financial or family distress<br>• Hopelessness and meaninglessness<br>• Guilt<br>• Fear of expressing anger<br>• Sleep deprivation | **Tricyclic Antidepressants** ***(continued)***<br>• Urinary retention, benign prostatic hypertrophy or intestinal motility present: use a drug with fewer anticholinergic effects (e.g., desipramine, nortriptyline)<br><br>**Psychostimulants**<br>• Rapid onset of action<br>• Energizing; reduces opioid-induced sedation<br>• Potential unwanted side effects: anxiety, insomnia, nightmares, psychosis, paranoia, tolerance<br>• Dosage: Give test dose at 8 am; reassess patient in 2 hours; discontinue medication if unwanted side effects occur<br>• Contraindications: hyperactive delirium or severe anxiety |

## Table 23. Some Pharmacological Agents for Treating Major Depression in Patients with Advanced Disease

| Drug | Initial Dose | Maximal Dose | Notes |
|---|---|---|---|
| **Serotonin-specific reuptake inhibitors** | | | Much less likely than tricyclics to alleviate neuropathic pain, but causes less sedation and dry mouth. Often reduces libido. |
| Citalopram (Celexa) | 10–20 mg | 60 mg | – Fewer drug interactions. Taper off when discontinuing |
| Paroxetine (Paxil) | 10 mg am | 50 mg | – May relieve diabetic neuropathic pain |
| Sertraline (Zoloft) | 50 mg am | 200 mg | – For frail elderly, begin with half the usual starting dose |
| **Newer Miscellaneous antidepressants** | | | Can be very useful for some patients with anxiety or low energy levels; cost may be a consideration. |
| Bupropion (Wellbutrin) | 100 mg PO bid | 300–450 mg/d | – Weak serotonin, norepinephrine, and dopamine reuptake inhibitor; useful for low energy; contraindicated with seizures, bulimia, anorexia. |
| Nefazodone (Serzone) | 50 mg bid | 300 mg bid | – Serotonin antagonist and reuptake inhibitor |
| Mirtazapine (Remeron) | 15 mg hs | 45 mg/d | – Norepinephrine and serotonin antagonist. Possible sedation, weight gain, agranulocytosis (0.1%) |
| Venlafaxine (Effexor) | 37.5 bid | 375 mg/d | – Available in sustained release<br>– Sometimes useful for neuropathic pain<br>– Low doses sedating, but higher doses activating |
| Seroquel / Quetiapine | 25 bid | | – 5HT + Dopamine |

*continued*

**Table 23. Some Pharmacological Agents for Treating Major Depression in Patients with Advanced Disease** *(continued)*

| Drug | Initial Dose | Maximal Dose | Notes |
|---|---|---|---|
| **Tricyclic antidepressants** | | | Best studied group. Helpful for insomnia and neuropathic pain. Give single dose, usually at bedtime. Has anticholinergic side effects, so increase slowly toward target dose, as tolerated. May need to monitor levels. |
| Amitriptyline (Elavil) | 10–75 mg PO HS | 300 mg | – Sedating; analgesic effects are well studied |
| Desipramine (Norpramin) | 10–75 mg PO HS | 300 mg | – Fewer side effects than amitriptyline; less sedating |
| Nortriptyline (Pamelor) | 10–25 mg PO HS | 150 mg | – Oral solution available |
| Doxepin (Sinequan) | 10–50 mg PO HS | 300 mg | – Sedating |
| **Psychostimulants** | | | Rapid effect, but may exacerbate anxiety and restlessness; taper off slowly if possible. |
| Methylphenidate (Ritalin) or Dextroamphetamine | 2.5 mg am and noon | 60 mg/d | – Doses greater than 30 mg/d are not usually necessary; occasionally, patients require up to 60 mg/d. |
| Pemoline (Cylert) | 18.75 mg am and noon | 75 mg/d | – Patients typically require no more than 75 mg/d; comes in chewable tablets that can be absorbed through the buccal mucosa; should be used with caution in patients with liver impairment. |
| **Benzodiazepine** | | | |
| Alprazolam (Xanax) | 0.25–1.0 mg tid | 4 mg/d | Helpful when anxiety coexists with depression. –Taper off slowly, if possible. |

## Table 24. Risk Factors for Suicide in Patients with Advanced Disease[48–50]

**Risk factors related to disease**

- Uncontrolled pain or other symptoms
- Advanced disease and poor prognosis
- Pharyngeal, lung, gastrointestinal, urogenital, or breast cancer
- Advanced HIV disease
- Exhaustion and fatigue

**Risk factors related to mental status**

- Depression and hopelessness
- Delirium and disinhibition
- Psychotic features (i.e., hallucinations and delusions)
- Loss of control, impulsiveness
- Irrational thinking
- Persistent suicidal ideation and lethal plans

**Risk factors related to personal and family history**

- Preexisting psychiatric disease (major depression, anxiety disorders)
- Substance abuse (alcohol)
- Recent loss (spouse or friends)
- Lack of social supports
- Older age, male sex
- Prior suicide attempts, family history of suicide
- Severe existential distress
- Fear of "being a burden"

## Table 25. Questions Reflecting Common Spiritual Issues

- Why am I here? Have I lived for nothing? Does my life have any meaning?
- Am I part of something larger than myself? Does a higher power such as God exist, and what is my relationship to that power?
- Why do I (or my loved one) have to suffer? Is suffering a punishment for something I've done? Am I to blame for the suffering of my loved ones? How can I find meaning in my current situation and transcend it?
- Why do I have to die? Does death have any meaning? What happens after I die?

## Table 26. Sample Definitions of Spirituality and Religion

**Spirituality**

- Spirituality is a broader, more inclusive category than religion. It can be defined as "that which allows a person to experience a sense of transcendence in life."[51] Spirituality is concerned with universal and ultimate issues of meaning and purpose in life, and with a person's relationship with all of reality, including the self, others, the natural world, the unexplainable mysteries of life and death, and, for some, a higher power.[52,53]
- Generally, spirituality is concerned with the ultimate *why* questions of existence.

**Religion**

- Religions are structured belief systems that address universal spiritual questions. They provide frameworks for making sense of ultimate questions of meaning. Their rites and rituals offer concrete ways of expressing spirituality.
- Because religious rituals and observances provide powerful sources of transcendence, inspiration, and comfort for many people, the religious beliefs of all terminally ill patients should be supported in every possible way, including making provisions for desired religious rituals and observances.

## Table 27. Principles of Spiritual Assessment

**Implications of the "spirituality-religion" relationship for palliative medicine**[54]

- A patient's expression of spirituality may or may not involve religion.
- Care plans should identify a patient's spiritual needs as well as religious concerns and needs.
- Interventions to alleviate spiritual pain should be based on the patient's belief system, whether or not it involves a specifically religious framework of meaning.

**Taking a spiritual history**[55]

- Consider spirituality a potentially important component of every patient's physical and emotional well-being. Take at least a brief spiritual history on every patient.
- Address spirituality at each complete physical exam, and address it at follow-up visits if appropriate. Spiritual growth is an on-going process that should receive greater attention when patients or their family members experience a life crisis, including a serious illness.

**Choosing language**

- Remember that although spirituality and religion are complementary concepts, they are not synonymous.
- Be cautious when using religion-specific language, discussing religious doctrines, or quoting religious texts. Listen carefully to patients and families. Take your cues from them, and respect and support what comforts them rather than what comforts you. For example, references to personal salvation are likely to offend members of non-Christian or liberal Christian traditions, as well as those whose belief systems are not based on a religious framework.
- Clichés such as "God never sends us more than we can bear," "Time heals all wounds," or "It is God's will," are examples of "theology by slogan" and are not helpful.[56] Avoid comments that may be interpreted as religious slurs, such as referring to a religious person as being "holier-than-thou."

**Responding to belief systems**

- Be aware of personal beliefs and biases. Some physicians or other members of a palliative/hospice team may become agitated or irritable when the subject of spirituality is raised, particularly when nondenominational or nontheistic approaches to spiritual assessment and intervention are suggested.[57] Clinicians may experience anxiety or distress when a patient's religious beliefs differ from their own or do not include the concept of a personal God or a higher power of any sort.
- Respect a patient's privacy regarding spiritual beliefs, and refrain from imposing your beliefs on others. Each patient's belief system should be honored and respected, whether it is religious, philosophical, or political in nature.
- In general, avoid discussions of specific religious doctrines, unless the patient indicates the doctrine is a particular source of spiritual pain or comfort. Individual beliefs vary tremendously, even between two people who share a common religious tradition.

*continued*

## Table 27. Principles of Spiritual Assessment *(continued)*

- The most appropriate response to patients' questions about the physician's religious beliefs is to help the patients find renewed hope and strength within their own belief systems. Inquire about past sources of strength and support and the use of religious or spiritual practices. (When physicians focus on their own religious beliefs, they may inadvertently interfere with the patient's own journey to transcendence and meaning.)
- Understand that integrating meaning into life is more important for spiritual healing than adherence to a particular belief system. When Elizabeth Kübler-Ross noted that good atheists die as well as good theists, she was trying to convey the message that both religious and nonreligious frameworks of meaning can provide strength and comfort for dying patients and their caregivers. Patients are likely to experience periods of great spiritual distress during the process of dying, regardless of their belief system or religious affiliation.[58]
- Be aware that your own spiritual beliefs can help you personally. Your beliefs affect your encounters with patients and can be used to make the doctor-patient encounter more caring and humanistic.
- Understand that for physicians working with dying patients and others with advanced disease, the most significant tasks of hospice/palliative medicine may be to increase the physician's awareness of personal beliefs and biases, develop tolerance for the beliefs and values of others, and deepen a personal sense of spirituality.[52]

**Encouraging spiritual healing**

- Each patient has the capacity to heal spiritually, but spiritual healing is more likely to occur when caregivers can identify the signs and symptoms of spiritual pain and provide interventions to alleviate specific sources of distress.
- Spiritual healing includes the following: acknowledging and then letting go of the anger, guilt, hurt, and fear that separate people from one another; finding ways of transcending the present situation, often by finding a sense of larger meaning in it; and opening to an enlarged sense of wholeness that transcends limiting roles and identities.
- Spiritual and religious practices can increase the capacity for spiritual healing.
- The path to spiritual healing begins with acknowledging spiritual pain.
- The approach of death can provide a powerful stimulus for spiritual healing.
- All religious traditions have developed teachings, practices, and rituals for facilitating spiritual healing.
- Interventions to alleviate spiritual pain rarely are neat and tidy. They involve at least two people—the physician and the patient—both of whom are struggling to enter into authentic relationship and find meaning in the present moment.

*continued*

## Table 27. Principles of Spiritual Assessment *(continued)*

**Finding meaning**

- Help patients formulate spiritual questions. Remember that exploring spiritual issues often is healing, even when no specific answers are revealed.
- Acknowledge the difficulty of coping with unanswerable questions, particularly when so much of medicine involves the skillful resolution of problems.
- Acknowledge and stay with the mystery of spirituality. Resist the temptation to explain death or tie the patient's spiritual pain into a tidy bundle of religious doctrine.
- Remember that achieving an intellectual understanding of meaning may be less important than experiencing a sense of peace and being at one with existence.
- Art, music, books, poetry, massage, prayer, meditation, and relaxation exercises may help the patient reach a sense of peace and unity that makes guilt about the past, concerns about the future, and less-than-perfect systems of meaning seem less significant.
- Be aware that, regardless of specific beliefs, continued presence and caring relationships give life and meaning to religious and philosophical abstractions about the importance of love.

**Responding to guilt and remorse**

- People often use alcohol, prescription drugs, or overactivity to avoid thinking about guilt, purpose, and meaning. When profound illness strikes, these methods of avoidance may no longer be available. Painful and long-repressed thoughts may intrude and cause suffering. If guilt focuses on specific actions, emphasize atonement and forgiveness rather than trivializing the guilt by making statements such as "You shouldn't feel that way."

**Establishing professional boundaries and making referrals**

- Referrals to chaplains, spiritual directors, or community resources should be made whenever appropriate and possible.
- Ethical questions have arisen concerning the actions of attending physicians who also wish to serve as pastoral caregivers.[59] Pressure to blur the professional boundary between serving as a medical caregiver and providing pastoral support may come from patients who want their physicians to pray with them. Unless a patient insists on physician-led prayer, religious rituals and observances usually are best provided by an identified religious leader. This approach avoids even the appearance of religious coercion on the part of the physician.[60]
- Physicians should be educated to understand spiritual concerns and to assess and identify spiritual pain, but it is important to delineate and respect professional boundaries between medical caregivers and professionals providing spiritual care.[59] The belief that anyone can provide intensive spiritual care trivializes the agony of deep spiritual pain.

## Table 28. FICA: A Spiritual Assessment Tool[55, 61]

| | |
|---|---|
| **F** | **Faith or Beliefs**<br>*Specific questions to elicit responses*<br>Do you consider yourself spiritual or religious? Both? Neither?<br>What things do you believe in that give meaning to your life?<br>What is your faith or belief? |
| **I** | **Importance and Influence of Beliefs**<br>*Specific questions to elicit responses*<br>Is your faith or belief important in your life?<br>What influence does your faith or belief have on how you take care of yourself?<br>How have your beliefs influenced your behavior during this illness?<br>What role do your beliefs play in regaining your health? |
| **C** | **Community**<br>*Specific questions to elicit responses*<br>Are you part of a spiritual or religious community?<br>Does the community provide support for you? How?<br>Is there a person or group of people you really love or who are really important to you? |
| **A** | **Address Care Issues**<br>*Specific questions to elicit responses*<br>How would you like me, as your healthcare provider, to address these issues while caring for you? |

Note: The FICA, developed by Christina Puchalski, MD, has been used to train more than 4,000 physicians. It can be effective regardless of a patient's system of belief and can help patients voice concerns about meaning and purpose in their lives, even when they don't recognize their concerns as being "spiritual." The assessment tool also can be used in a time-constrained setting, where 2 minutes may be all that is allotted for a spiritual history, especially during a routine visit. Puchalski MC, Rorner AL. Taking a spiritual history allows clinicians to understand patients more fully. *J Palliat Med.* 2000; 3: 129–137. Copyright, Christina M. Puchalski, MD, 1996. Adapted and reprinted with permission from Christina M. Pulchaski, MD. For more information, contact the George Washington Institute for Spirituality and Health (www.gwish.org).

## Table 29. Three Dimensions of Spiritual Need[53]

**Situational transcendence:** In this dimension, patients want to make sense of and transcend their current situation. They often desire

- purpose
- hope
- meaning and affirmation
- mutuality
- a sense of connection
- social presence

**Moral and biographical transcendence:** In this dimension, patients want to "put things right," to make sense of their own lives, and to develop a sense of transcendent meaning for their existence. They often desire

- peace and reconciliation
- reunion with others
- prayer
- moral and social analysis
- forgiveness
- closure

**Religious transcendence:** In this dimension, patients want to achieve a sense of religious transcendence. They often desire

- religious reconciliation
- divine forgiveness and support
- religious rites or sacraments
- visits by clergy
- religious literature
- discussion about God, eschatology, or eternal life and hope

## Table 30. Interventions to Alleviate Spiritual Pain[52]

**Alleviating spiritual pain related to individual and community needs**

- Control physical symptoms (pain, anxiety, depression) that exacerbate spiritual pain.
- Provide supportive presence.
- Encourage life review.
- Explore issues of guilt, blame, remorse, forgiveness, and reconciliation.
- Explore the nature and cause of the breakdown of the patient's spiritual support system. Support ways to strengthen the patient's past spiritual support systems.
- Support meaningful relationships with significant others.

**Alleviating spiritual pain related to need for general meaning**

- Encourage reflection on past, current, or desired belief systems, philosophies, or world views.
- Encourage practical application of the patient's belief system or philosophy to the current situation.
- Identify elements of past or current belief system or philosophy that provided support in the past. Encourage reestablishment of those elements.
- Explore the patient's religious history as a cause of pain. Some patients may feel terribly wounded by the religion of their childhood and need to come to terms with their anger and sense of rejection.
- Encourage patients to tell their life stories as a way of helping them recognize themes of purpose, value, worth, and meaning. (See *UNIPAC Two: Alleviating Psychological and Spiritual Pain in the Terminally Ill.*)

**Alleviating spiritual pain related to religious needs**

- Observe the patient's special holy days, dietary restrictions, need for daily prayer or meditation, hygiene and modesty requirements, and other important religious precepts.
- Remember the power of religious rituals and observances and, when appropriate, provide or arrange for the following:
  - prayers that focus on healing and reconciliation
  - sacraments of baptism, confirmation, marriage, and reconciliation; sacrament of the sick
  - ritualized confession, reconciliation, absolution of sins, asking for forgiveness
  - laying on of hands
  - devotional practices (e.g., meditation, prayer, turning toward Mecca, reading religious scriptures from sources such as the Hebrew and Christian bibles, the Bhagavad-Gita, and the Koran)

*continued*

**Table 30. Interventions to Alleviate Spiritual Pain[52] *(continued)***

| |
|---|
| **Alleviating spiritual pain related to inner resource needs**<br>• Help patients identify elements in the past that have given meaning to their lives and helped them feel more alive and empowered (e.g., use of spiritual or religious practices, contact with nature, relationships, meaningful communication with significant others).<br>• Encourage life review and exploration of sources of meaning in life.<br>• If the patient desires, arrange for access to books or meditation tapes to enhance inner resources.<br>• Encourage use of adaptive techniques such as relaxation, imagery, music, poetry, and devotional readings that focus on healing rather than cure. If the patient desires, arrange for access to spiritual or religious teachers who use meditation, prayer, and religious scriptures to focus on healing instead of physical cures.<br>• Help patients reframe goals into short-term tasks that can be accomplished, such as going on a trip or saying good-bye to friends and family. |

## Table 31. Herth Hope Index©[62]

**Listed below are a number of statements. Read each statement and place an X in the box that describes how much you agree with that statement *right now*.**

| | Strongly Disagree | Disagree | Agree | Strongly Agree |
|---|---|---|---|---|
| 1. I have a positive outlook toward life. | | | | |
| 2. I have short, intermediate, and/or long-range goals. | | | | |
| 3. I feel all alone. | | | | |
| 4. I can see a light in a tunnel. | | | | |
| 5. I have faith that gives me comfort. | | | | |
| 6. I feel scared about my future. | | | | |
| 7. I can recall happy/joyful times. | | | | |
| 8. I have deep inner strength. | | | | |
| 9. I am able to give and receive caring/love. | | | | |
| 10. I have a sense of direction. | | | | |
| 11. I believe that each day has potential. | | | | |
| 12. I feel my life has value and worth. | | | | |

**Scoring:**

All items except numbers 3 and 6 are scored as follows:
Strongly disagree = 1; Disagree = 2; Agree = 3; Strongly agree = 4
Items 3 and 6 are reverse scored as follows:
Strongly disagree = 4; Disagree = 3; Agree = 2; Strongly agree = 1

No specific score indicates whether or not a person has adequate hope. However, comparing a patient's responses over time can reveal important information. Discussing the results of each completed index provides an opportunity for professional caregivers to gently probe selected issues with patients and discuss possible interventions, including reframing hope during the course of a terminal illness.

Farran CJ, Herth KA, Popovich JM. *Hope and Hopelessness: Critical Clinical Contructs.* Thousand Oaks, CA: Sage Publications, Inc; 1995. Reprinted with permission from Kaye A. Herth, who developed the Herth Hope Index and retains the copyright. Permission to use or reproduce the Herth Index must be obtained from KA Herth.

## Table 32. Strategies for Fostering Hope in Patients, Families, and Medical Staff[63]

**Provide comfort and relieve suffering.**

- Effectively control pain and other distressing symptoms (See *UNIPAC Three: Assessment and Treatment of Pain in the Terminally Ill*[3] and *UNIPAC Four: Management of Selected Non-pain Symptoms in the Terminally Ill.*[4]).
- Acknowledge and address all causes of suffering.

**Develop caring relationships.**

- Develop caring relationships with others (e.g., patients, family members, and professional caregivers).
- Relationships that include a sense of being needed and being part of something larger are particularly important.

**Set attainable goals and involve patients in decision making.**

- Recognize the small joys of the present, develop a sense of purpose or direction that fosters a sense of meaning in life, and redefine aims as needed. As physical deterioration becomes more evident, the patient's aims are likely to gradually change from accomplishing specific tangible aims, to more global aims that include hopes for the well-being of other people, to a sense of "being" rather than "having or doing" that includes hope for such things as serenity, inner peace, and eternal rest or life.

**Support spirituality.**

- Many terminally ill patients express belief in God or some other higher power, but some do not. Regardless of specific religious beliefs, recognize that a spiritual base can provide a sense of meaning and security that transcends human explanation.
- Support the use of meaningful religious rites and rituals when requested.

**Identify valued personal attributes and affirm the patient's worth.**

- Acknowledge that personal attributes such as determination, courage, and serenity can help patients and others maintain hope.
- Treat people as dignified, worthwhile human beings.
- Recognize that affirmations of worth and treatment as a valued and worthwhile person can help a patient, family member, or healthcare professional maintain hope.

*continued*

## Table 32. Strategies for Fostering Hope in Patients, Families, and Medical Staff[63] *(continued)*

**When appropriate, use lighthearted humor.**

- Healthcare professionals may be the only ones with whom patients can laugh about their situation. Patients often appreciate verbal or nonverbal expressions of delight, joy, or playfulness from professional staff (when appropriate and when patients trust that staff will also listen to their deepest concerns). After a physician has earned a patient's trust and demonstrated concern, empathy, and respect for the patient's condition, humor and lightheartedness, when appropriate, can provide a sense of release from thoughts and fears about the disease and can bring joy and hope to a darkened room.
- Family members may need to be reminded that laughter can be very helpful.
- For more information on the appropriate use of humor, see *UNIPAC Five: Caring for the Terminally Ill: Communication and the Physician's Role on the Interdiscplinary Team.*[5]

**Reminisce about life, and emphasize uplifting memories.**

- Recalling pleasant moments by sharing happy stories, looking at photograph albums, and reminiscing about significant events such as the birth of a child can help maintain hope.

# 3. Assessment and Management of Pain

## Assessing Pain

The four components of total pain are listed in **Table 33**, page 60. See **Table 34**, page 61, for principles of pain assessment. See **Table 35**, pages 62–63, for information on identifying pain syndromes.

## Pain Assessment Tools

Using developmentally appropriate assessment scales is a critical component of managing pain and other symptoms, particularly when patients are unable to verbalize discomfort. Scales should be completed by the patient whenever possible and be simple enough to use regularly. The same scale should be used consistently with the patient. Scales also are useful for assessing the effectiveness of an intervention, for assessing an entire program's symptom relief efforts, and for gathering data for research projects.[66] See **Table 36**, pages 64–65, for a pain assessment tool for adults. See **Table 104**, page 159, and **Figures 5–7**, page 161, for scales for children. See *UNIPAC Three: Assessment and Treatment of Pain in the Terminally Ill, 2nd ed, Hospice and Palliative Medicine Self-Study Progran for Physicians,*[3] and *UNIPAC Eight: The Hospice and Palliative Medicine Approach to Caring for Pediatric Patients*[8] for more information on assessment scales.

## Treating Pain

### Nonpharmacologic Interventions

#### *Physical Interventions*

See **Table 37**, page 66, for physical interventions for treating generalized weakness and the aches and pains commonly associated with a cancer diagnosis and therapy. Physicians should encourage patients to remain active and to participate in self-care as long as possible.

#### *Cognitive-Behavioral Interventions*

See **Table 38**, pages 67–69, for cognitive-behavioral interventions that can increase a patient's sense of control and enhance skills for coping with pain. Cognitive-behavioral interventions are *not* substitutes for effective pharmacologic interventions.

## Pharmacologic Interventions: WHO Analgesic Ladder

The World Health Organization (WHO) Analgesic Ladder (**Figure 3**, page 70) illustrates a simple three-step approach to pain management based on the type of analgesia required to effectively control pain of increasing intensity.

See **Table 39**, page 71, for principles of analgesic use.

## Nonsteroidal Antiinflammatory Analgesics

See **Table 40**, pages 72–77, for nonsteroidal antiinflammatory analgesics.

## Opioids

See **Table 41**, pages 78–79, for equianalgesic and opioid starting doses for opioid-naïve adults and children. See **Table 42**, page 80 for conversion of some oral opioid doses to parenteral doses.

## Titrating Opioids

See **Table 43**, page 81, for guidelines for opioid titration. **Table 44**, page 81, lists examples of titration increments for opioid dosing.

## Adjuvant Analgesics for Treating Pain Syndromes

See **Table 45**, pages 82–84, for suggested adjuvant drugs and dosages for treating pain syndromes in adults.

## Titrating Adjuvant Drugs in Patients with Liver Disease and Renal Failure

### *Patients with Liver Disease*

Liver disease has the greatest effect on drugs that undergo extensive oxidative metabolism. Liver disease should have no effect on the disposition of drugs excreted unchanged by the kidneys. No useful noninvasive test of liver function exists to guide dosage adjustments—typical liver function tests reflect but do not predict the extent of liver damage. See **Table 46**, pages 85–86, for examples of dosage adjustments in patients with liver disease. For more information, see *UNIPAC Three: Assessment and Treatment of Pain in the Terminally Ill.*[3]

### *Patients with Renal Failure*

Because many medications and their metabolites are metabolized and/or excreted by the kidneys, individualized pharmacologic dosing is important in patients with renal impairment. Renal failure also can contribute to the development of electrolyte, acid-base, vascular volume, nutritional, and hematologic problems. Renal failure can either increase or decrease the volume of distribution of certain drugs, thus affecting their metabolism. Acid-base changes occurring with renal failure can affect protein binding, thus altering bound and unbound levels of medications and their metabolites. Be aware of age-related declines in renal function in the elderly.

Measurements of creatinine clearance ($CL_{CR}$) are helpful when determining appropriate medication dosing in patients with renal disease. The following are easy methods for estimating creatinine clearance:

- For males: $CL_{CR}$ = (140-age)Weight (in kilograms) divided by 72 x Serum creatinine
- For females: $CL_{CR}$ = $CL_{CR}$male x 0.85

See **Table 47**, pages 87–89, for examples of dosage adjustments in patients with renal failure. See *UNIPAC Three: Assessment and Treatment of Pain in the Terminally Ill*[3] for more information.

### Managing Refractory Pain

See **Table 48**, page 90, for information on managing refractory pain.

### Methadone

**Table 49**, page 91, illustrates one method of rotating opioids to oral or rectal methadone.

### Invasive Interventions

See **Table 50**, pages 92–93, for examples of invasive interventions.

## Drugs and Routes to Avoid in Hospice/Palliative Care Settings

See **Table 51**, page 94 for drugs and routes to avoid in hospice/palliative care settings.

**Table 33. Four Components of Total Pain**

| | |
|---|---|
| **P** | Physical problems, often multiple, must be specifically diagnosed and treated.[64] |
| **A** | Anxiety, anger, and depression are critical components of pain that must be recognized and addressed by the physician, in conjunction with other health-care professionals. |
| **I** | Interpersonal problems, including loneliness, financial stress, and family tensions, which are often interwoven in the fabric of a patient's symptoms, must be addressed. |
| **N** | Nonacceptance of approaching death, a sense of hopelessness, and a desperate search for meaning in life can cause severe spiritual suffering unrelieved by medications. |

*Notes*

1. All components of total pain—physical pain, social pain, emotional pain, and spiritual pain—interact with each other. If unrelieved, each component contributes to total pain or suffering.
2. Assessments should include a history, physical, and use of a numerical or visual analogue pain assessment scale, which encourages patients to share information about a pain's location, intensity, and etiology.

## Table 34. Principles of Pain Assessment

- Complete a careful history and physical. Performing a complete assessment is the essential first step of pain management, because it provides the foundation for effective control of pain.
- Use open-ended questions, and listen carefully to what the patient says.
- Use developmentally appropriate pain assessment scales completed by the patient (whenever possible) to determine the site, intensity, and quality of each pain.
- Assess for pain caused by noncancer-related conditions (e.g., arthritis, decubiti, migraine headaches, muscle strain, oral thrush, surgery, injuries).
- Assess for psychosocial and spiritual pain caused by emotional, social, and spiritual factors (e.g., anxiety, depression, loneliness, loss of meaning, financial concerns).
- Assess for cancer-related pain.[65]
  - direct tumor involvement (78%) (e.g., bone metastases, nerve compression/infiltration, hollow viscus, visceral organs)
  - cancer therapy (19%) (e.g., surgery, radiotherapy, chemotherapy, medication side effects [constipation, urinary retention, etc.])
  - pain unrelated to cancer or cancer therapy (3%) (e.g., arthritic pain, post-herpetic neuralgia)
- Reassess at regular intervals, after initiation of each new treatment, after each new report of pain or change in the quality/intensity of pain, and at appropriate intervals after pharmacologic or nonpharmacologic interventions.[65]
- Treat pain empirically while investigating its etiology.[65]

## Table 35. Identifying Pain Syndromes in Cancer

### Somatic/ Tissue and Bone Pain

- Mechanism: activation of nociceptors (e.g., bone metastases, muscle/soft tissue tumor infiltration)
- Character of pain
  - constant or intermittent
  - usually gnawing, aching
  - occasionally cramping
  - well localized
- Drug therapy: Bone pain is partially responsive to opioid therapy but may require anti-inflammatory drugs, steroids, or other adjuvants or radiotherapy for adequate relief. (See Table 45, pages 82–84.)

### Visceral Pain

- Mechanism: activation of nociceptors (e.g., intra-abdominal or liver metastases)
- Character of pain
  - constant
  - aching, squeezing, cramping
  - poorly localized, occasionally referred, occasionally well localized
- Drug therapy: Opioid analgesics and possibly anticholinergics or octreotide (See Table 45, pages 82–84.)

### Neuropathic Pain

Mechanism: Destruction/infiltration/compression of nerve tissue. Neuropathic pain generally presents in two clinical manifestations:

*Dysesthetic Pain (deafferentation pain)*

- Character of pain
  - constant burning
  - occasionally radiates (e.g., post-herpetic pain)
- Primary drug therapy: Opioids + tricyclic antidepressants (Anticonvulsants also may be needed.) (See Table 45, pages 82–84.)

*continued*

**Table 35. Identifying Pain Syndromes in Cancer** *(continued)*

*Neuralgic Pain*

- Character of pain
  - paroxysms of lancinating pain
  - sharp, shooting pain (e.g., trigeminal neuralgia)
- Primary drug therapy: Opioids + anticonvulsants, tricyclic antidepressants, or other adjuvants (See Table 45, pages 82–84.)

*Breakthrough or Incident Pain*

- Mechanism: Activation of nociceptors in weight-bearing bones of soft tissues upon movement. Psychological stress also can heighten sensitivity to pain.
- Character of pain
  - dramatic increase or movement, weight bearing, or stress
- Therapy
  - immobilization with orthopedic surgery or splinting
  - bolus analgesia before movement (e.g., IV/SC opioid or transmucosal fentanyl [Actiq])

## Table 36. Brief Pain Assessment Inventory (Short Form)[67]

**Date:** _____/_____/_____

**Time:** __________

**Name:** ________________________________________

Last First Middle Initial

1. Throughout our lives, most of us have had pain from time to time (such as minor headaches, sprains, and toothaches). Have you had pain other than these everyday kinds of pain today? 1. Yes 2. No
2. On the diagram, shade in the areas where you feel pain. Put an X on the area that hurts the most.

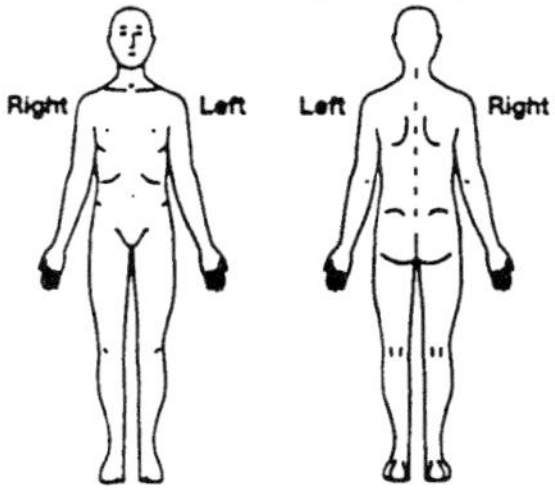


3. Please rate your pain by circling the one number that best describes your pain at its worst in the past 24 hours.

   0 1 2 3 4 5 6 7 8 9 10

   No pain Pain as bad as you can imagine

4. Please rate your pain by circling the one number that best describes your pain at its least in the past 24 hours.

   0 1 2 3 4 5 6 7 8 9 10

   No pain Pain as bad as you can imagine

5. Please rate your pain by circling the one number that best describes your pain on the average.

   0 1 2 3 4 5 6 7 8 9 10

   No pain Pain as bad as you can magine

6. Please rate your pain by circling the one number that best tells how much pain you have right now.

   0 1 2 3 4 5 6 7 8 9 10

   No pain Pain as bad as you can imagine

*continued*

**Table 36. Brief Pain Assessment Inventory (Short Form)[67]** *(continued)*

7. What treatments or medications are you receiving for your pain?

8. In the past 24 hours, how much relief have pain treatments or medications provided? Please circle the one percentage that most shows how much relief you have received.

   10% 20% 30% 40% 50% 60% 70% 80% 90% 100%
   Little relief Complete relief

9. Please circle the one number that describes how, during the past 24 hours, pain has interfered with your:

   A. General activity
   0 1 2 3 4 5 6 7 8 9 10
   Does not interfere Completely interferes

   B. Mood
   0 1 2 3 4 5 6 7 8 9 10
   Does not interfere Completely interferes

   C. Walking ability
   0 1 2 3 4 5 6 7 8 9 10
   Does not interfere Completely interferes

   D. Normal work (includes both work outside the home and housework)
   0 1 2 3 4 5 6 7 8 9 10
   Does not interfere Completely interferes

   E. Relations with other people
   0 1 2 3 4 5 6 7 8 9 10
   Does not interfere Completely interferes

   F. Sleep
   0 1 2 3 4 5 6 7 8 9 10
   Does not interfere Completely interferes

   G. Enjoyment of life
   0 1 2 3 4 5 6 7 8 9 10
   Does not interfere Completely interferes

Source: Pain Research Group, Department of Neurology, University of Wisconsin-Madison. May be duplicated and used in clinical practice.

## Table 37. Physical Interventions for Controlling Pain[68]

**Cutaneous Stimulation.** Noninvasive techniques can be taught to the patient or caregiver.

- ***Heat.*** Avoid burns by wrapping the heat source (e.g., hot pack or heating pad) in a dry towel. Lying on an electric heating pad can result in burns. The use of heat on irradiated tissue is contraindicated. Diathermy and ultrasound are not recommended for use over tumor sites.
- ***Cold.*** Apply flexible ice packs that conform to body contours for periods not to exceed 15 minutes. Cold treatment provides longer lasting relief than heat but should not be used by patients with peripheral vascular disease or on tissue damaged by radiation therapy.
- ***Massage, pressure, and vibration.*** These methods, which help the patient through distraction or relaxation, sometimes increase pain before relief occurs. Massage should not be substituted for exercise in ambulatory patients.

**Exercise.** Useful for treating subacute and chronic pain; strengthens weak muscles; mobilizes stiff joints; helps restore coordination and balance; enhances patient comfort; and provides cardiovascular conditioning. Therapists and trained family members or other caregivers can help functionally limited patients with range-of-motion exercises to preserve strength, joint function, and mobility. During acute pain, exercise should be limited to self-administered range of motion. Weight-bearing exercise should be avoided if bones are likely to fracture.

**Repositioning.** Reposition the immobilized patient frequently to maintain correct body alignment, alleviate pain, and help prevent pressure ulcers.

**Immobilization.** Use restriction of movement to manage acute pain or to stabilize fractures or otherwise compromised limbs or joints. Use adjustable elastic or thermoplastic braces to help maintain correct body alignment. Keep joints in position of maximal function rather than maximal range. Avoid prolonged immobilization.

### Counterstimulation

- ***Transcutaneous electrical nerve stimulation (TENS).*** Controlled, low-voltage electrical stimulation applied to large myelinated peripheral nerve fibers via cutaneous electrodes to inhibit pain transmission. Although the efficacy of TENS can be partially attributed to a placebo effect, patients with mild pain may benefit from a trial of TENS.
- ***Acupuncture.*** Pain treated by inserting small, solid needles into the skin. Multiple randomized controlled trials have demonstrated its efficacy in the control of dental pain, and evidence suggests efficacy in other painful conditions and some nonpain symptoms such as nausea.[69] Acupuncture should only be attempted by a skilled professional. Because pain can signal disease progression, infection, or treatment complications, patients should be encouraged to report new pain problems to the healthcare team prior to using acupuncture.

*Note:* Noninvasive physical interventions can be used concurrently with drugs and other interventions to manage pain during all phases of treatment. The effectiveness of physical interventions depends on the patient's participation and ability to communicate the method(s) that best alleviate pain.

## Table 38. Cognitive-Behavioral Interventions for Controlling Pain[68,70]

**Relaxation and Imagery**

Simple relaxation techniques can be used during episodes of brief pain (e.g., during procedures) and when the patient's ability to concentrate is compromised by severe pain, high levels of anxiety, or fatigue. During exercises 1 and 3, the caregiver should speak clearly and calmly, pausing when appropriate.

***Relaxation Exercises***

*Exercise 1. Slow rhythmic breathing for relaxation*

Step 1. Breathe in slowly and deeply.

Step 2. As you breathe out slowly, feel yourself beginning to relax; feel the tension leaving your body.

Step 3. Now breathe in and out slowly and regularly, at whatever rate is comfortable for you. You may wish to try abdominal breathing.

Step 4. To help focus on your breathing and to breathe slowly and rhythmically (a) breathe in as you say silently to yourself, "in, two, three"; (b) breathe out as you say silently to yourself, "out, two, three." Or, each time you breathe out, say silently to yourself a word such as "peace" or "relax."

Step 5. Do steps 1–4 only once or repeat steps 3 and 4 for up to 20 minutes.

Step 6. End with a slow deep breath. As you breathe out say to yourself, "I feel alert and relaxed."

*Exercise 2. Simple touch, massage, or warmth for relaxation*

- Brief touch or massage (e.g., holding the patient's hand or briefly touching or rubbing the patient's shoulder)
- Warm foot soak in a basin of warm water, or feet wrap in a warm, wet towel
- Massage (3–10 minutes) may consist of whole body massage or be restricted to back, feet, or hands. If the patient has special concerns about modesty or cannot move or turn easily in bed, consider massaging the hands and feet.

  – Use a warm lubricant. (A small bowl or bottle of hand lotion may be warmed briefly in a microwave oven or in a sink of hot water.)

  – Massage for relaxation is usually done with smooth, long, slow strokes. (Rapid strokes, circular movement, and squeezing of tissues tend to stimulate circulation and increase arousal.) Try several degrees of pressure along with different types of massage (e.g., kneading, stroking, and circling to determine which type the patient prefers).

*continued*

## Table 38. Cognitive-Behavioral Interventions for Controlling Pain[68,70] *(continued)*

*Exercise 3. Peaceful past experiences*

In the past, something may have happened to you that brought you a sense of peace and comfort. You may be able to draw on that past experience to bring you a sense of peace and comfort now. Think about these questions:

1. Can you remember any situation, even when you were a child, when you felt calm, peaceful, secure, hopeful, or comfortable?
2. Have you ever daydreamed about something peaceful? What were you thinking of?
3. Do you get a dreamy feeling when you listen to music? Do you have any favorite music?
4. Do you have any favorite poetry that you find uplifting or reassuring?
5. Have you ever been religiously active? Do you have favorite readings, hymns, or prayers? Even if you haven't heard or thought of them for many years, childhood religious experiences may still be soothing.

Additional points: Some of the things you think about in answer to these questions can be recorded for you; for example, your favorite music or a prayer. You can listen to the tape whenever you wish. Or, if your memory is still strong, you may simply close your eyes and recall the events or words.

*Exercise 4. Active listening to recorded music*

1. Obtain the following:
   - A cassette player or tape recorder (Small, battery-powered ones are more convenient.)
   - Earphone or headset (This provides more stimulation than a speaker and avoids disturbing others.)
   - Cassette of music the patient likes (Most people prefer fast, lively music but some select relaxing music. Other options are comedy routines, sporting events, old radio shows, or stories.)
2. Patient can mark time to the music (e.g., tap out the rhythm with finger or nod head). This promotes concentration on music rather than discomfort.
3. Patient can keep eyes open and focus steadily on one stationary spot or object or close eyes and picture something about the music.
4. Patient can listen to the music at a comfortable volume. If discomfort increases, try increasing the volume; decrease the volume when the discomfort decreases.
5. If this is not effective enough, try adding or changing one or more of the following techniques: patient can massage own body in rhythm to the music; try other music; mark time to the music in more than one manner (e.g. tap foot and finger at the same time).

*continued*

## Table 38. Cognitive-Behavioral Interventions for Controlling Pain[68,70] *(continued)*

**Cognitive Distraction and Reframing**

Cognitive distraction focuses attention on stimuli other than on the pain or the negative emotions accompanying pain. Techniques include internal distractions (e.g., counting, praying, or making self-statements such as "I can cope."), or external distractions (e.g., music, television, talking, listening to someone read). Cognitive reframing involves learning to monitor and evaluate negative thoughts and replacing them with more positive thoughts and images.

**Patient Education**

Patient education should emphasize that almost all pain can be effectively managed. Oral and written information should address pain and symptom assessment and treatment, including pharmacologic and other interventions used to control symptoms. Major barriers to effective pain management should be addressed to correct misconceptions about pain and symptom management.

**Psychotherapy and Structured Support**

Some patients benefit from short-term psychotherapy provided by psychotherapists. Patients who develop symptoms of clinical depression or other adjustment disorders should be referred to professionals with training in psychotherapy. The relationship between poorly controlled pain, depression, and thoughts of suicide should not be ignored.

**Support Groups and Pastoral Counseling**

Clinicians should be aware of locally active peer support groups and provide information to patients and their families. Members of the healthcare team who specialize in pastoral counseling should participate in team discussions and provide information on community resources for spiritual support of the patient and family.

*Note:* The interventions are more likely to succeed when introduced early in the course of illness, giving patients time to become proficient while they still have enough energy to practice. Patients and families should try several strategies, then select one or two that are particularly helpful.

**Figure 3. World Health Organization Analgesic Ladder**

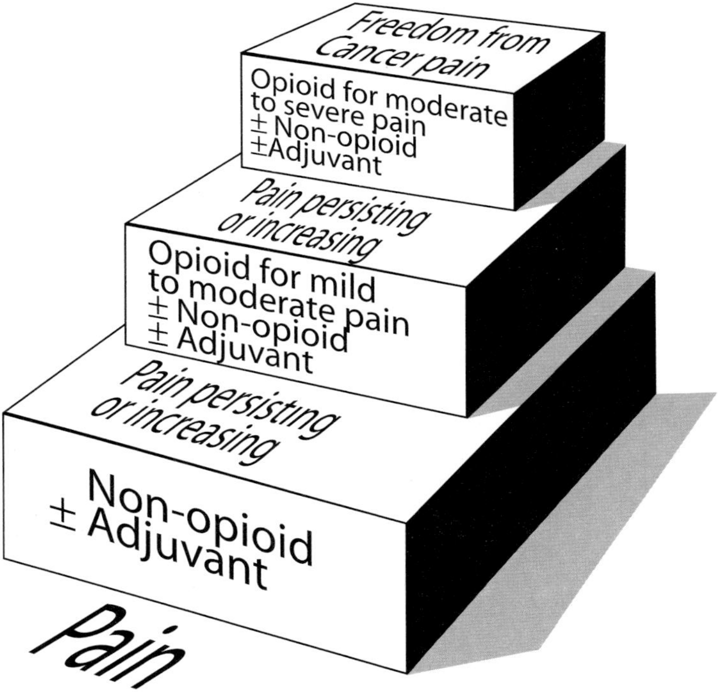


Reprinted with permission of World Health Organization, from *Cancer Pain Relief*, 2nd ed. Geneva, 1996.

## Table 39. Principles of Analgesic Use

| | |
|---|---|
| **By the mouth** | The oral route is the preferred route for analgesics, including morphine. |
| **By the clock** | Persistent pain requires around-the-clock treatment to prevent further pain. PRN dosing is irrational and inhumane; it requires patients to experience pain before becoming eligible for relief. |
| **By the WHO ladder** | If a maximum dose of medication fails to adequately relieve pain, move up the ladder, not laterally to a different drug in the same efficiency group. Severe pain requires immediate use of an opioid recommended for controlling severe pain, without progressing sequentially through Steps 1 and 2. |
| **Individualize treatment** | The right dose of an analgesic is the dose that relieves pain with acceptable side effects for a specific patient. |
| **Monitor** | Monitoring is required to ensure the benefits of treatment are maximized while adverse effects are minimized. |
| **Use adjuvant drugs** | For example, an NSAID is almost always needed to help control bone pain. Non-opioid analgesics, such as NSAIDs or acetaminophen, can be used at any step of the ladder. Adjuvant medications also can be used at any step to enhance pain relief or counteract the adverse effects of medications (see Table 45, pages 82–84.)[10,71] |

**Table 40. Nonsteroidal Antiinflammatory Analgesics**

| Generic Name | Approximate Half-Life (Hours) | Dosing Schedule (Hours) | Starting Dose (mg/d)[1] Adults >50 kg |
|---|---|---|---|
| **Paraaminophenol Derivatives** | | | |
| Acetaminophen (Tylenol) | 2–4 | q 4–6 | 2,600 mg |
| **Salicylates** | | | |
| Acetylsalicylic acid[3] (aspirin) | 3–12 | q 4–6 | 3,750 mg |
| Choline magnesium trisalicylate (Trilisate) | 8–12 | q 8–12 | Initial dose: 1,500 mg, then 1,500 mg q 8–12 hours |
| Diflunisal (Dolobid) | 8–12 | q 12 | Initial dose: 1,000 mg, then 500 mg q 12 hours |
| Salsalate (Disalcid) | 8–12 | q 12 | Initial dose: 1,500 mg, then 1,500 mg q 12 hours |
| **Propionic Acids** | | | |
| Flurbiprofen (Ansaid) | 5–6 | q 8–12 | 100 mg |
| Ibuprofen (Motrin, Advil, Nuprin) | 2–4 | q 4–8 | 400–600 mg q 6–8 hours |
| Ketoprofen (Orudis) | 2–4 | q 6–8 | 25–50 mg q 8 hours in mild renal impairment and elderly. 75 mg q 8 hours or 50 mg q 6 hours |
| Naproxen (Naprosyn) | 13 | q 12 | 500 mg |
| Naproxen sodium (Anaprox, Aleve) | 13 | q 12 | 550 mg |

| Maximum Dose (mg/d)[3] | Excretion | Comments |
|---|---|---|
| 4,000 mg | 85% renal | Lacks peripheral antiinflammatory and antiplatelet effect. Excessive dosing → liver toxicity. Monitor platelet and liver function with chronic disease. Adults and children >50 kg: 10–15 mg/kg q 4 hours. |
| 6,000 mg | 100% renal | May inhibit platelet aggregation for >1 week. Contraindicated in children with fever or other viral syndromes. |
| 4,500 mg | 100% renal | Approved for children. Minimal gastrointestinal toxicity. Suspension available. See note 2. |
| 1,000 mg | 90% renal, <5% fecal | |
| 3,000 mg | 100% renal | See note 2. |
| 300 mg | 65%–85% renal | |
| 3,200 mg | 50%–75% renal | Suspension formulation available. |
| 300 mg | 50%–90% renal, 1%–8% fecal | |
| 1,500 mg | 95% renal | |
| 1,100 mg | 95% renal | |

*continued*

**Table 40. Nonsteroidal Antiinflammatory Analgesics** *(continued)*

| Generic Name | Approximate Half-Life (Hours) | Dosing Schedule (Hours) | Starting Dose (mg/d)[1] Adults >50 kg |
|---|---|---|---|
| **Propionic Acids** *(continued)* | | | |
| Oxaprozin (Daypro) | 50–60; 40 with repeated dosing | q 24 | 1,200 mg |
| **Acetic Acids** | | | |
| Diclofenac (Voltaren) | 2 | q 6 | 100 mg |
| Indomethacin (Indocin, Indocide, Indomethine) | 4–5 | q 8–24 | 75 mg |
| Sulindac (Clinoril) | 8–16 | q 12 | 300 mg |
| Tolmetin (Tolectin) | 1 | q 8 | 1,200 mg |
| **Oxicam** | | | |
| Piroxicam (Feldene) | 50 | q 25 | 20 mg |
| **Fenamates** | | | |
| Meclofenamic acid (Meclomen) | 50 minutes–3.3 hours | q 4–6 | 50–100 mg |
| Mefenamic acid (Ponstel) | 2 | q 6 | Loading dose: 500 mg, then 250 mg |
| **COX-2 Inhibitors** | | | |
| Celecoxib (Celebrex) | 11 | q 12 | 100 mg bid |
| Rofecoxib (Vioxx) | 17 | q 24 | 12.5 mg |
| Valdecoxib (Bextra) | 8–11 | q 24 | 10 mg |
| **Pyrrolo-pyrrole** | | | |
| Ketorolac (Toradol) | 4–6 | q 4–6 | IV/IM 30–60 mg loading dose, then 1/2 loading dose q 6 hours; PO 10 mg q 6 hours |

| Maximum Dose (mg/d)[3] | Excretion | Comments |
|---|---|---|
| 1,800 mg | 60% renal, 30%–35% fecal | |
| 200 mg | 50%–70% renal, 30%–35% fecal | |
| 200 mg | 60% renal, 30% fecal | Available in sustained release and rectal formulations. Greater gastrointestinal and central nervous system toxicity. See note 3. |
| 400 mg | 50% renal, 25% fecal | |
| 1,800 mg | 100% renal | |
| 40 mg | 67% renal, 33% fecal | Progressive increase in response may occur because of long half-life. Steady state 7–12 days after initiation of therapy. |
| 400 mg | 67% renal, 20%–25% fecal | Dose-related diarrhea. |
| 1,000 mg | 67% renal, 33% fecal | Intended for short-term use. Dose-related diarrhea. |
| 400 mg | 97% hepatic metabolism, 3% renal | Less gastrointestinal toxicity. Higher cost. See note 2. |
| 50 mg | 99% hepatic metabolism, 1% renal | Less gastrointestinal toxicity. Higher cost. See note 2. |
| 20 mg | Renal | Less gastrointestinal toxicity. Higher cost. See note 2. |
| 120 mg IV/IM; 40mg PO | 91% renal, 6% fecal | Short-term use only (5 days). |

*continued*

**Table 40. Nonsteroidal Antiinflammatory Analgesics** *(continued)*

| Generic Name | Approximate Half-Life (Hours) | Dosing Schedule (Hours) | Starting Dose (mg/d)[1] Adults >50 kg |
|---|---|---|---|
| **Pyranocarboxylic acids** | | | |
| Etodolac (Lodine) | 6–7 | q 6–8 | 200–400 mg |
| **Naphthylalkanones** | | | |
| Nabumetone (Relafen) | 23–30 | q 12–24 hours | 1,000 mg |

*Notes*

1. Starting and maximal dosages are not intended to preclude clinical judgment of the prescribing clinician. Dosage reduction recommended for elderly, renal insufficiency, multiple medications. Initial doses usually may be titrated upward. Doses can be incremented weekly. Studies of nonsteroidal antiinflammatory drugs (NSAIDs) in the cancer population are limited-dosing guidelines are based on studies in inflammatory diseases, thus doses in cancer patients are empiric.
2. Minimal platelet effects.

| Maximum Dose (mg/d)[3] | Excretion | Comments |
|---|---|---|
| 1,200 mg | 60% renal, 27% fecal | |
| 2,000 mg | renal | A pro-drug. Gastrointestinal and kidney toxicity may be less common. |

## Table 41. Equianalgesic and Opioid Starting Doses for Opioid-Naïve Adults and Children

| Drug | Equianalgesic Dose Oral (Compared to 30 mg PO Morphine ) | Usual Starting Dose PO <50 kg | Usual Starting Dose PO >50 kg | PO:IV/SC Ratio |
|---|---|---|---|---|
| Codeine | 190 mg ("usual" maximum dose is 120 mg) | 0.5–1 mg/kg q 3–4 hours | 15-30 mg q 3–4 hr | 1.5:1.0 SC **Not to be given IV.** |
| Hydrocodone (as in Vicodin) | 30 mg (Clinical experience suggests lower potency.) | 0.1 mg/kg q 3–4 hours | 5–10 mg q 3–4 hr | Not available in parenteral form |
| Oxycodone (as in Percocet, Tylox) | 20 mg | 0.1–0.2 mg/kg q 3–4 hours | 5–10 mg q 3–4 hr | Not available in parenteral form |
| Morphine | 30 mg | 0.15–0.3 mg/kg q 3–4 hours | 5–10 mg q 3–4 hr | 3:1 |
| Hydromorphone (Dilaudid) | 7.5 mg | 0.05 mg/kg q 3–4 hours | 1-2 mg q 3–4 hr | 5:1 |
| Oxymorphone (Numorphan) | N/A | N/A | N/A | 5 mg PR equianalgesic with 1 mg IV |
| Fentanyl Intravenous (Caution-Rapid infusion may cause chest wall rigidity) | N/A | N/A | N/A | N/A |

NA = not available TD = Transdermal

*Notes*

1. When converting from one short half-life opioid to another, reduce the dose of the new opioid by 25%–50% of the equianalgesic dose (because of incomplete cross-tolerance), then titrate as required.
2. Usual starting doses often are empiric and NOT necessarily calculated according to equianalgesic principles (e.g., the usual starting dose for hydromorphone may be 2 mg PO even though the parenteral: oral ratio = 1:5).
3. For infants <6 months of age, use 1/4 of the usual starting dose, then titrate to effect.
4. Transdermal fentanyl not recommended for use in opioid-naïve patients.
5. Conversion to a long-acting preparation is recommended after dose titration achieves pain relief.

Modified from Memorial Sloan-Kettering Cancer Center Pain Service

| Equianalgesic Dose Parenteral (Compared to 10 mg IV Morphine) | Usual Starting Dose IV/SC <50 kg | >50 kg | Biologic Half-Life (Hours) |
|---|---|---|---|
| 130 mg (usual maximum dose is 60 mg) | 0.25–0.5 mg/kg q 3–4 hr SC **Not to be given IV.** | 60 mg Q 3–4 hrs SC. **Not to be given IV.** | 2.5–3 |
| N/A | N/A | N/A | 3–4 |
| N/A | N/A | N/A | 2–3 |
| 10 mg | 0.05–0.1 mg/kg q 3–4 hr | 5–10 mg q 3–4 hr | 2.5–3 |
| 1.5 mg | 0.02–0.07 mg/kg q 3–4 hr | 1–1.5 mg q 3–4 hr | 2–3 |
| 1 mg | 0.02 mg/kg q 3–4 hr | 1 mg q 3–4 hr | 1.5 |
| **Single dose**: 100 mcg **By infusion:** 100 mcg/h = 2.5 mg/h morphine | 0.5–1.5 mcg/kg q 30 min | 25–75 mcg q 30 min | IV: 3–12 hours TD: 18–24 hours (elimination half-life) TD:IV Ratio=1:1 (Based on clinical experience) |

## Table 42. Conversion of Oral Opioid Doses to Parenteral Doses

| Drug | PO | SC or IV |
|---|---|---|
| Morphine | 20 mg → | divide by 3 → 7 mg |
| | 20 mg → | divide by 20 → 1 mg |
| Hydromorphone | 5 mg → | divide by 5 → 1 mg |

## Table 43. Guidelines for Opioid Titration

- Titrating opioids to effectively control pain is an important pain management technique. No ceiling or maximal recommended opioid dose exists—the effective dose is the correct dose. Large doses of morphine (e.g., several hundred milligrams every 4 hours) may be needed to relieve severe pain.[72]
- Immediate-release morphine is a 4-hour drug that reaches its peak effect in approximately 1 hour when delivered orally, and in 10–20 minutes when delivered subcutaneously. When pain is not relieved within peak times of the administration of a higher dose, additional doses should be given.
- During the titration process, no ceiling exists on the number of times a dose may be titrated. Over a 24-hour period, some patients may require more than a 100% increase over their initial daily baseline dose. See Table 44 for examples of recommended titration increments.
- When titrating opioids, continuing reassessment is needed to identify
  - pain that does not respond to opioids (i.e., pain that requires treatment with adjuvant drugs or other specific remedies).
  - nonphysical pain that requires treatment with compassionate listening and the involvement of other members of the interdisciplinary team. *See UNIPAC Two: Alleviating Psychological and Spiritual Pain in the Terminally Ill.*[2]

## Table 44. Examples of Titration Increments for Opioid Dosing*

| Baseline 4-Hour Dose (mg) | Titration Increment (mg) (1/2 of 4-hour dose or 10% of daily dose) |
|---|---|
| 1–10 | 1–5 |
| 10–20 | 5–10 |
| 20–30 | 10–15 |
| 40–50 | 20–25 |
| 100 | 30–50 |
| 200 | 50–100 |
| 500 | 100–250 |
| 1,000 | 250–500 |

*The increment doses also are appropriate for use as "rescue doses" when breakthrough pain occurs. (For more information, see *UNIPAC Three: Assessment and Treatment of Pain in the Terminally Ill.*[3])

## Table 45. Suggested Adjuvant Drugs and Dosages for Treating Pain Syndromes in Adults

***Somatic, Tissue, and Bone Pain***

| Pain Character | Drug Class | Examples | Notes |
|---|---|---|---|
| Tenderness over bone or joint on movement | NSAIDs | See Table 40, pages 72–77. | |
| | Bisphosphonates | Pamidronate (Aredia) 60–90 mg diluted in 500–1,000 mL of N/S and given IV over 4–6 hours | For bone metastases or Paget's disease. Cannot be administered SC, may exacerbate renal insufficiency. |
| | Steroids | Dexamethasone 2–8 mg bid to qid PO or SC | Adverse effects of long-term administration are well known. Potential early side effects: loss of glucose control, increased risk of infection, acute psychiatric disorders (e.g., mania). |

***Neuropathic Pain:*** An antidepressant and an anticonvulsant may be needed. In difficult cases, check for therapeutic serum levels of both the antidepressant and the anticonvulsant.

| Pain Character | Drug Class | Examples | Notes |
|---|---|---|---|
| Continuous burning or tingling, pain on light touch | Tricyclic antidepressants | Amitriptyline (Elavil) 10–50 PO mg q hs | Best studied, sedating, start with low dose, anticholinergic effects. |
| | | Doxepin (Sinequan)10–50 mg PO q hs | 10 mg/cc suspension available. If patient unable to swallow, insert capsules rectally (50 mg q 12 hours). |
| | | Trazodone (Desyrel) 25–150 mg PO q hs | Less anticholinergic effect, 1/3 as potent as amitriptyline, sedating. |
| | | Nortriptyline (Pamelor) 10–50 mg PO q hs | Less anticholinergic effect. Suspension available. |

*continued*

**Table 45. Suggested Adjuvant Drugs and Dosages for Treating Pain Syndromes in Adults** *(continued)*

***Neuropathic Pain*** *(continued)*

| Pain Character | Drug Class | Examples | Notes |
|---|---|---|---|
| Shooting, stabbing pain | Anticonvulsants | Gabapentin (Neurontin) 100–300 mg PO qhs and increase rapidly as tolerated | Effective but costly. |
| | | Valproate (Depakote) 250 mg PO tid–qid | Both carbamazepine and valproate are absorbed from the rectum. |
| | | Carbamazepine (Tegretol) 200 mg PO q 6–12 hours | Start at lower dose if pain is not severe. Liquid form available. If patient unable to swallow, crush tablets, put in gelatin capsules, and give rectally (600 mg q 6–8 hours) |
| | | Clonazepam (Klonopin) 0.5 mg PO bid–qid or 0.01 mg/kg initially | Sedating |
| | | Phenytoin (Dilantin) 300-400 mg PO qd or load with15–20 mg/kg IV (in a crisis) | Rarely first line |
| | Local anesthetics | Mexiletine (Mexitil) 150 mg bid–qid or 1 mg/kg in bid–tid doses; may require up to 900 mg/d | GI side effects<br>Monitor EKG and/or blood levels as appropriate. |
| | | Lidocaine SC or IV infusion | Monitor EKG |
| | | Lidocaine transdermal 5% (Lidoderm) | Apply to painful areas. |
| | | Lidocaine/prilocaine topical (Emla) | Apply to painful areas. |
| | Other agents | Clonidine 0.1–0.3 mg PO bid or clonidine transdermal (Catapres-TTS) 0.1–0.3 mg/24 hours | Monitor blood pressure, watch for rebound hypertension, depression, bradycardia. |

*continued*

**Table 45. Suggested Adjuvant Drugs and Dosages for Treating Pain Syndromes in Adults** *(continued)*

***Neuropathic Pain*** *(continued)*

| Pain Character | Drug Class | Examples | Notes |
|---|---|---|---|
| | | Baclofen 5–20 mg PO tid | Watch for drowsiness, dizziness. |
| | | Calcitonin nasal spray (Miacalcin) | Delayed onset of analgesia, few side effects. |
| | | Capsaicin topical (Zostrix) 0.025 or 0.075% cream apply tid–qid. | Commonly causes burning sensation and thermal hyperalgesia. |

***Visceral Pain***

| Pain Character | Drug Class | Examples | Notes |
|---|---|---|---|
| Colic, camping abdominal pain, bladder spasms | Anticholinergics | Scopolamine (Transderm Scop) 1–2 patches q 3 days | |
| | | Hyoscyamine (Levsin) 0.125 mg PO or SL q 4–8 hours | Available as sublingual tablet, liquid, sustained-release preparation |
| | | Oxybutynin (Ditropan) 5–10 mg PO q 8 hours | Tablets or liquid |
| | Steroids | Dexamethasone 4 mg PO/SC qd–tid | Can relieve a partial bowel obstruction. If no benefit in 5 days, discontinue. |

## Table 46. Examples of Dosage Adjustments in Patients with Liver Disease[73,74]

| Medication | Hepatic Elimination | Dosage Adjustment |
|---|---|---|
| **Adjuvants** | | |
| Carbamazepine | >98% hepatic | Decrease dose |
| Dexamethasone | >97% hepatic | Decrease dose |
| Phenytoin | >95% hepatic | Decrease dose in severe disease |
| Mexiletine | 90% hepatic | Decrease dose by 60–70% |
| Prednisone | >85% hepatic | None |
| **Analgesics** | | |
| Acetaminophen | >95% hepatic | Avoid chronic use* |
| Fentanyl | 92% hepatic | None |
| Ibuprofen | >99% hepatic | Decrease dose in severe disease* |
| Methadone | 80% hepatic | None or decrease* |
| Morphine | 90% gastrointestinal and hepatic | Decrease dose or use a different opioid |
| Naproxen | >90% hepatic | Decrease dose in severe disease |
| Propoxyphene | >95% gastrointestinal and hepatic | Decrease by 50%* |
| **Antidepressants** | | |
| Amitriptyline | Primarily hepatic | Use with caution |
| Fluoxetine | Primarily hepatic | Decrease by 50% |
| Nefazodone | Primarily hepatic | Decrease dose |
| **Antiemetics** | | |
| Metoclopramide | 80% hepatic | Decrease by 50%* |
| Ondansetron | >95% hepatic | Decrease frequency in severe disease |

*continued*

## Table 46. Examples of Dosage Adjustments in Patients with Liver Disease[73,74] *(continued)*

| Medication | Hepatic Elimination | Dosage Adjustment |
|---|---|---|
| **Antihistamine** | | |
| Diphenhydramine | >98% hepatic | Decrease dose |
| **Anxiolytics** | | |
| Alprazolam | >90% hepatic | Decrease by 50% |
| Chlordiazepoxide | >99% hepatic | Decrease* |
| Diazepam | >97% hepatic | Chronic, decrease dose* |
| Lorazepam | >98% hepatic | None |
| Midazolam | >95% hepatic | Decrease dose by 50% |
| **Diuretics** | | |
| Bumetanide | 36% hepatic | None |
| Furosemide | 35% hepatic | None |
| Hydrochlorothiazide | <10% hepatic | None |
| Spironolactone | >85% hepatic | None |
| Triamterene | >95% hepatic | Decrease dose |
| **Gastrointestinal** | | |
| Cimetidine | 40% hepatic | Decrease dose in severe disease* |
| Famotidine | 30% hepatic | None* |
| Omeprazole | >90% hepatic | Decrease dose by 50% |
| Ranitidine | 30% hepatic | None* |
| **Sedative/Hypnotics** | | |
| Temazepam | >98% hepatic | None |
| **Other** | | |
| Pamidronate | 30% hepatic | None |

*In hepatic failure, choose an alternative agent.

## Table 47. Examples of Dosage Adjustments for Patients with Renal Failure[75–77]*

| Medication | Adjustment For Renal Failure ($CL_{CR}$)* | |
|---|---|---|
| | 10–50 ml/min | <10 ml/min |
| **Adjuvants** | | |
| Amitriptyline | 100% | 100% |
| Carbamazepine | 100% | 100% |
| Desipramine | 100% | 100% |
| Dexamethasone | 100% | 100% |
| Mexiletine | 100% | 50%–75% |
| Nortriptyline | 100% | 100% |
| Phenytoin | 100% | 100% |
| Prednisone | 100% | 100% |
| Gabapentin | q 12–24 hours | qod |
| **Analgesics** | | |
| Acetaminophen | q 6 hours dosing | q 8 hours dosing |
| Codeine | 75% | 50% |
| Diclofenac | 25%–50% | 25% |
| Fentanyl | 100% | 100% |
| Ibuprofen | 100% | 100% |
| Ketorolac | 50% | 25%–50% |
| Methadone | 100% | 50%–75% |
| Morphine | 75% | 50% |
| Naproxen | 100% | 100% |
| Propoxyphene | 100% | Avoid |
| Acetylsalicylate | q 4–6 hours dosing | Avoid |
| Sulindac | 100% | 100% |
| **Antidepressants** | | |
| Amoxapine | 100% | 100% |
| Bupropion | 100% | 100% |
| Fluoxetine | 100% | 100% |
| Sertraline | 100% | 100% |
| **Antiemetics** | | |
| Cisapride | 100% | 50% |
| Haloperidol | 100% | 100% |

*continued*

**Table 47. Examples of Dosage Adjustments For Patients With Renal Failure**[75–77*] *(continued)*

| Medication | Adjustment For Renal Failure ($CL_{CR}$)* 10-50 ml/min | <10 ml/min |
|---|---|---|
| **Antiemetics** *(Continued)* | | |
| Granisetron | 100% | 100% |
| Metoclopramide | 75% | 50% |
| Ondansetron | 100% | 100% |
| Prochlorperazine | 100% | 100% |
| **Antihistamines** | | |
| Diphenhydramine | 100% | 100% |
| Hydroxyzine | 50% | 50% |
| **Anxiolytics** | | |
| Alprazolam | 100% | 100% |
| Chlordiazepoxide | 100% | 50% |
| Clonazepam | 100% | 100% |
| Diazepam | 100% | 100% |
| Midazolam | 100% | 50% |
| Oxazepam | 100% | 100% |
| **Bronchodilators** | | |
| Albuterol | 75% | 50% |
| Terbutaline | 50% | Avoid |
| Theophylline | 100% | 100% |
| **Diuretics** | | |
| Bemetadine | 100% | 100% |
| Furosemide | 100% | 100% |
| Spironolactone | q 12–24 hours dosing | Avoid |
| Thiazides | 100% | Avoid |
| Triamterene | q 12 hours dosing | Avoid |
| **Gastrointestinal** | | |
| Cimetidine | 50%–75% | 25%–50% |
| Famotidine | 25%–50% | 10% |
| Misoprostil | 100% | 100% |
| Omeprazole | 100% | 100% |

*continued*

**Table 47. Examples of Dosage Adjustments for Patients with Renal Failure**[75-77]* *(continued)*

| Medication | Adjustment For Renal Failure ($CL_{CR}$)* 10-50 ml/min | <10 ml/min |
|---|---|---|
| **Gastrointestinal** *(Continued)* | | |
| Ranitidine | 50% | 25% |
| Sucralfate | Avoid | Avoid |
| **Hypoglycemic Agents** | | |
| Acarbose | Avoid | Avoid |
| Glipizide | 50% | 50% |
| Glyburide | 100% | 100% |
| Insulin | 75% | 50% |
| **Inotropic Agents** | | |
| Dobutamine | 100% | 100% |
| Milrinone | 100% | 50%–75% |
| **Sedative/Hypnotics** | | |
| Flurazepam | 100% | 100% |
| Phenobarbital | 100% | 100% |
| Temazepam | 100% | 100% |
| Triazolam | 100% | 100% |
| **Other** | | |
| Chlorpromazine | 100% | 100% |
| Warfarin | 100% | 100% |

*100% means that no dosage adjustment is required.

## Table 48. Managing Refractory Pain

- Look for reversible causes (e.g., constipation, urinary retention, infected wounds, unstable fractures).
- Look for neuropathic pain (burning, shooting, or exquisitely tender to light touch).
  - Consider a loading dose of an anticonvulsant. (See Table 45, pages 82–84.)
  - Consider a trial of IV or SC lidocaine (1–5 mg/kg over 20–60 minutes) followed by PO mexiletine. (See Table 45, pages 82–84.)
- Consider rapid dose escalation of a potent opioid and/or a change to IV or SC infusion.
- Consider rotating the opioid to methadone, which can be very effective for relieving pain in selected patients with pain uncontrolled by large doses of conventional opioids such as morphine and hydromorphone. Local toxicity when using the SC route is controllable with site rotation and dexamethasone infused concurrently with the methadone.[78] Methadone has proven to be particularly useful for treating severe pain when high doses of other opioids result in unacceptable side effects.[79] Methadone can be administered PO, IV, PR, or SC (with dexamethasone or hyaluronidase).[80] The process of converting from other opioids to methadone is complex due to its long half-life. Conversion requires considerable attention, experience, and usually 3–6 days in an inpatient setting, where patients' highly variable reactions can be monitored closely.[81] The dose ratio of methadone to morphine or hydromorphone changes according to the total opioid dose. See Table 49 for the method used at the Palliative Care Unit in Edmonton, Canada.
- Consider a consultation with an anesthesiology pain specialist for a trial of ketamine, an epidural or intrathecal infusion of an opioid plus bupivacaine or clonidine, or a neurolytic block.
- Consider more invasive interventions (See Table 50, page 92).

## Table 49. One Method of Rotating Opioids to Oral or Rectal Methadone[82]

**Day 1**

- Decrease previous opioid dose by 1/3.
- Replace with 3% of previous daily oral morphine equivalent dose, given as oral or rectal methadone every 8 hours (e.g., a patient receiving 1000 mg of oral morphine is switched to 660 of oral morphine + 30 mg/d of oral methadone 10 mg PO or PR q 8 hours)

**Day 2**

- Decrease previous opioid by another 1/3, *if* pain is controlled with rescue doses of a short-acting opioid.
- Increase methadone dose only if pain is moderate to severe.

**Day 3**

- Discontinue final 1/3 of previous opioid.
- For breakthrough pain, give patient a rescue dose of about 10% of the daily methadone dose, orally or rectally.
- Continue daily assessment of pain and dose titration until reaching an effective stable dose of methadone.

Adapted from Bruera E, Neumann CM. Role of methadone in the management of pain in cancer patients. *Oncology.* 1999;13(9):1275–1282.

## Table 50. Examples of More Invasive Interventions[68]

**Radiation Therapy**

- Local or whole-body radiation enhances the effectiveness of analgesic drug therapy and other noninvasive therapies by directly affecting the cause of pain (i.e., reducing the primary and metastatic tumor bulk). A dosage must be chosen that achieves a balance between the amount of radiation required to kill tumor cells and that which adversely effects normal cells or prohibits the repair of damaged tissue. Single or reduced fraction treatments often are effective for long-bone metastases.
- A single intravenous injection of beta particle–emitting agents such as iodine-131, phosphorus-31-orthophosphate, strontium-89, rhenium-186, and samarium-153 can relieve pain caused by widespread bony metastases. If pain recurs, 50% of patients respond to a second treatment. Single-dose treatments are better tolerated by frail terminally ill patients.

**Surgery**

Curative excision or palliative debulking of a tumor can reduce pain directly, relieve symptoms of obstruction or compression, and improve prognosis. The potential benefits and burdens of surgery (including pain syndromes that follow specific surgical procedures) should be carefully considered in light of the patient's goals of care and expected prognosis. In many cases, pharmacologic management of the symptoms of bowel obstruction and other conditions meet a terminally ill patient's goals of care more effectively than surgery.

**Nerve Blocks**

Control of otherwise intractable pain can be achieved with a relatively brief application of a local anesthetic or neurolytic agents. Nerve blocks can be considered when pain is not controlled with other interventions, even when provided by physicians with expertise in palliative medicine. When managing cancer pain, nerve blocks are performed for several reasons:

- diagnostic: to determine the source of pain (e.g., somatic versus sympathetic pathways) This course is likely to be unduly burdensome for a terminally ill patient.
- therapeutic: to treat painful conditions that respond to nerve blocks (e.g., celiac block for pancreatic cancer pain)
- prognostic: to predict the outcome of long-lasting interventions (e.g., infusion, neurolysis, rhizotomy)
- preemptive: to prevent painful sequelae of procedures that may cause phantom limb, causalgia, or reflex sympathetic dystrophy

*continued*

## Table 50. Examples of More Invasive Interventions[68] *(continued)*

**Nerve Blocks** *(continued)*

- A single injection of a nondestructive agent such as lidocaine or bupivacaine, alone or in combination with an antiinflammatory corticosteroid for a longer-lasting effect, can provide local relief from nerve or root compression. Placement of an infusion catheter at a sympathetic ganglion extends the sympathetic blockade from hours to days or weeks. Destructive agents such as ethanol or phenol can be used to effect peripheral neurolysis at sites identified by local anesthesia as appropriate for permanent pain relief.

**Neurosurgery**

Like neurolytic blockage, ablation of pain pathways should be reserved for situations when other therapies are ineffective or poorly tolerated. Devices can be implanted to deliver drugs or to electrically stimulate neural structures. Generally, the choice of neurosurgical procedure is based on the location and type of pain (somatic, visceral, deafferentation), the patient's general condition and life expectancy, and available expertise and follow-up.

**Epidural or Spinal Infusions**

An anesthesiologist often can insert a temporary catheter into the epidural or subarachnoid space to deliver an opioid or a combination of an opioid and a local anesthetic. Much smaller doses are usually required, and side effects can be minimal. The addition of clonidine can help relieve neuropathic pain. If effective, a more permanent catheter can be tunneled subcutaneously for outpatient use. Complications include kinked or dislodged catheters and serious infections.

Note: With rare exceptions (e.g., radiation therapy to prevent a long-bone fracture or spinal cord compression), less invasive interventions should precede invasive palliative measures. In the small minority of patients for whom behavioral, physical, and pharmacologic interventions do not relieve pain, invasive therapies may be useful.

## Table 51. Drugs and Routes to Avoid in Hospice/Palliative Care Settings

| | |
|---|---|
| **Drug** | |
| Meperidine (Demerol) | • Very low potency.<br>• Toxic metabolite accumulation. |
| Pentazocine (Talwin) | • No more potent than codeine.<br>• High incidence of hallucinations and agitation (30% in cancer patients).<br>• Inhibits analgesia of morphine. |
| **Route** | |
| IM Injection | • Morphine 30 mg PO is as potent as 10 mg IM/SC.<br>• Avoid the pain and expense of injections by using PO or SC morphine.<br>• If a patient cannot tolerate anything PO, start a SC infusion or give slow-release morphine tablets rectally. |

# 4. Management of Nonpain Symptoms

## Prevalence of Symptoms

See **Table 52**, page 97, for information on symptom prevalence in patients with cancer.

## Emergent Conditions

Physicians must maintain a high index of suspicion for emergent conditions that require immediate and aggressive treatment. See **Table 53**, pages 98-101, for examples of emergent conditions.

## Anorexia/Cachexia

See **Table 54**, page 102, for steps to manage anorexia and cachexia.

## Anxiety

For information on anxiety and depression, see Chapter 2 and *UNIPAC Two: Alleviating Psychological and Spiritual Pain in the Terminally Ill*.[2]

## Bowel Obstruction

See **Table 55**, page 103, for medical management of bowel obstruction.

## Cognitive Impairment and Delirium

### Cognitive Impairment

Simple and sensitive screening tests for cognitive impairment include the Mini-Mental State Examination (MMSE) and clock drawing. *Clock drawing* involves asking the patient to draw a clock, either freely or one that reads ten minutes after eleven o'clock. The degree of aberration in the drawing tends to correlate with the degree of disturbance in executive function. The *MMSE* is a well-validated, widely used tool for screening for cognitive impairment in many population groups, including patients with advanced disease. It is brief, easy to administer by clinical staff or lay personnel, and measures orientation to time and place, immediate recall, short-term memory, ability to calculate, attention and recall, and language.[88, 89]

## Delirium

See **Table 56**, pages 104–105, for information on assessment, family education, and general treatment of delirium. See **Table 57**, page 106, for treatment of moderate to severe agitated delirium.

## Depression

For information on anxiety and depression, see Chapter 2 and *UNIPAC Two: Alleviating Psychological and Spiritual Pain in the Terminally Ill.*[2]

## Constipation

See **Table 58**, page 107, for causes, symptoms, and treatments for constipation.

## Cough

See **Table 59**, page 108, for the etiology and treatment of cough.

## Diarrhea

See **Table 60**, page 109, for causes and treatments of diarrhea.

## Dysphagia

See **Table 61**, pages 110–111, for causes and treatments of dysphagia.

## Dyspnea

See **Table 62**, page 112, for specific causes and treatments for dyspnea and **Table 63**, page 113, for general measures for treating dyspnea.

### Opioid Therapy for Dyspnea

When no treatable etiology can be identified or when the general and specific treatments already mentioned do not completely alleviate the distressing symptoms associated with dyspnea, opioids are first-choice treatment agents because they suppress respiratory awareness so effectively. For information on using opioids to treat dyspnea, see **Table 64**, page 114. When individually titrated, opioids have been shown repeatedly to be safe and effective in the treatment of dyspnea caused by cancer.[100] In patients with chronic obstructive pulmonary disease, opioids decrease breathlessness and increase exercise tolerance with decreased ventilation.[101]

To treat dyspnea, order the same opioids on the same schedules as those prescribed for pain, and increase the dose every 4–12 hours until the patient is comfortable. See **Table 65**, page 115, for information on managing refractory dyspnea.

## Fatigue

**Table 66**, page 115, details proposed criteria for fatigue in cancer and other progressive illnesses. For management of fatigue, see **Table 67**, page 116.

## Hiccups

See **Table 68**, page 117, for causes and treatments of hiccups.

## Nausea/Vomiting

See **Table 69**, pages 118–119, for causes and treatments of nausea. See **Table 70**, pages 120–122, for pharmacologic management. See **Table 71**, page 123, for managing refractory nausea.

## Pruritus

See **Table 72**, page 124, for assessment and management of pruritus.

## Respiratory Secretions

See **Table 73**, page 125, for assessment and management of respiratory secretions.

## Refractory Symptoms

See **Table 74**, page 125, for assessment and management of refractory pain and other symptoms.

**Table 52. Symptom Prevalence in Patients with Cancer[83,84]**

| | Prevalence % | | |
|---|---|---|---|
| Symptom | Edmonton Palliative Care Service, Canada | St. Christopher's Hospice, UK | Memorial Sloan-Kettering Cancer Center, USA |
| Asthenia | 90 | 91 | 74 |
| Anorexia | 85 | 76 | 44 |
| Pain | 76 | 62 | 64 |
| Nausea | 68 | 44 | 44 |
| Constipation | 65 | 51 | 35 |
| Sedation/ confusion | 60 | N/A | 60 |
| Dyspnea | 12 | 51 | 24 |

## Table 53. Management of Emergent Conditions[85,86]

### Cardiac Tamponade

- Common causes include tumor spread to lungs or mediastinum.
- Occurs most commonly with cancers of lung and breast, lymphomas, or leukemias.
- Symptoms include chest pain, dyspnea, cough, orthopnea, weakness, and dizziness.
- Exam reveals pulsus paradoxus, hypotension, muffled heart sounds, friction rub, or tachycardia. Chest radiograph reveals new cardiomegaly, and electrocardiogram shows low voltage or electrical alternans. Echocardiogram is diagnostic.

### Delirium

- Acute confusional state often due to a medical condition.
- Look for
  - dehydration
  - hypercalcemia
  - psychotropic medication
  - failure of lungs, heart, kidneyss, or liver

### Hemorrhage, massive

- Head and neck tumors are more likely to infiltrate large vessels and vascular structure, leading to catastrophic exsanguination.

### Hypercalcemia

- 80% of all cases of hypercalcemia are caused by production of the parathyroid hormone-like peptide.
- A minority of cases are due to direct bone destruction, although bone metastatic lesions are a common cause of hypercalcemia in patients with malignancy.
- The main desired outcome of treating hypercalcemia is improvement in symptoms.
- Correction of calcium is not expected to improve cognitive failure that precedes hypercalcemia.
- Hypercalcemia: corrected calcium is >2.65 mmol/L (or 10.6 mg/dL).
- Look for
  - nausea and vomiting
  - dehydration
  - somnolence
  - confusion
  - polyuria, polydipsia
  - lethargy/weakness
  - irritability/agitation

## Factors to Consider

- Pericardiocentesis provides rapid relief.
- Pericardial windows or drainage and sclerosis prevent recurrence.
- If patient is close to death, treatment focuses on symptom control with analgesics, anxiolytics, and oxygen.

---

- See Tables 56 and 57, pages 104–105, and 106.

---

- Anticipate and sensitively instruct the patient, family, and caregivers on emergency administration of a sedative for the patient (e.g., midazolam 2.5 mg–5 mg SC prn, titrated to effect
- Use dark towels to absorb blood and apply pressure to site if hemorrhaging is external

---

- Treat hypercalcemia if the patient is symptomatic and has an adequately long prognosis.
- Adjust the serum calcium according to the serum albumin. Corrected serum calcium = measured serum calcium + [(40-measured serum albumin) x 0.02]. For example, a patient's measured calcium level is 2.4 mmol/L and the serum albumin is 20. Therefore, the corrected serum calcium is 2.4 + [(40-20) x 0.02] = 2.4 + 0.4 = 2.8 mmol/L.
  Note: The traditional U.S. measurement of mg/dl is four times larger than mmol/L. Therefore, 2.4 mmol/L = traditional U.S. measurement of 9.6 mg/dL and 2.8 mmol/L = 11.2 mg/dL.
- A one-time dose of a bisphosphonate is usually adequate. Bisphosphonates can exacerbate renal failure. Prior to administering a bisphosphonate, assess renal function (urea + creatinine blood levels). If prerenal azotemia is present (blood urea nitrogen >20 x creatinine), rehydrate the patient with normal saline prior to administering bisphosphonate.

### Mild hypercalcemia

- If dehydrated, rehydrate with normal saline, e.g., hypodermoclysis or IV at 100 mL/h or IV at 100–120 mL/h. In a small number of cases, this alone is sufficient. A diuretic such as furosemide may be needed.

### Moderate to severe hypercalcemia

- Pamidronate 60–90 mg diluted in 500–1,000 mL of normal saline, given IV over 4–6 hours. Cannot be given SC.
- Clodronate 1,500 mg diluted in 500–1000 mL of normal saline and given IV over 4–6 hours. Not currently available in the United States.

*continued*

Zometa

## Table 53. Management of Emergent Conditions[85,86] *(continued)*

**Hypercalcemia** *(continued)*

**Pain, Uncontrolled**

**Seizures**
- Occur most often in patients with cerebral tumors or meningeal involvement; less often in patients with metabolic disturbances, infection, drug toxicity, drug withdrawal, intracerebral hemorrhages.

**Spinal Cord Compression**
- Occurs in about 5% of patients with cancer.
- Early diagnosis and treatment are important if function is to be preserved. The most important determinant of neurological outcome is the degree of impairment when treatment is started.
- Delay in treatment may result in paralysis and bowel and bladder incontinence.
- Look for
  - central back pain, aggravated by movement coughing, or straining
  - progressive weakness and sensory loss
  - motor weakness
  - reduced rectal tone
  - nerve root irritation at the site of vertebral involvement
  - urinary retention, loss of bowel control
  - reduced reflexes

**Superior Vena Cava Syndrome**
- Onset is typically gradual, and usually originates from tumor in right, upper mediastinum.
- Typically from lung cancer, lymphomas, and metastatic cancer to lungs.
- Symptoms include hoarseness due to vocal cord edema, headache from cerebral edema, cough and dyspnea.
- On exam, look for facial plethora, facial and upper extremity edema as well as dilated collateral veins over chest wall, distention of arm veins that is unrelieved when arms are lifted.

(Case reports indicate clodronate can be administered SC. Suggested dose is clodronate 1,500 mg diluted in 1,000 mL of normal saline given SC over 12 hours.)

- Calcitonin is a temporary option for patients with severe symptoms needing rapid reduction in symptoms while being hydrated or treated with bisphosphonate. Consider calcitonin 100–200 U tid SC x 3–6 doses.
- Dexamethasone 4–8 mg PO/SC/IV bid may also be useful.

- See Chapter 3 on managing pain and especially Table 48, page 90.

**Management of acute seizure**

- Diazepam 10 mg IV if already IV access, or 10 mg PR using the parenteral solution
  OR
- Lorazepam 2 mg IV, SL, or SC
- Fosphenytoin (CEREBYX) 15 mgPE /kg IV, then 4–6 mgPE/kg/d by IV/SC infusion (PE = phenytoin equivalents)

**For patients unable to swallow**

**Continuing prophylaxis**

- Phenobarbital 120 mg (or 2 mg/kg) SC qd–tid (very sedating)
- Clonazepam 1–5 mg/d by continuous SC infusion
- Phenytoin 15–20 mg/kg up to 1 g IV, then 5–8 mg/kg/d in 2 doses IV
- Midazolam 5–30 mg/d by SC infusion

**If the patient is ambulatory, consider:**

- Immediate referral to confirm diagnosis (with computed tomography or magnetic resonance imaging scan) and initiate therapy (radiotherapy, occasionally surgery)
- Dexamethasone 6–10 mg tid to qid, as soon as diagnosis made or strongly suspected.

- Initial symptom management with elevation of head and avoidance of venipunctures and IV access in upper extremities.
- Steroids (dexamethasone) may reduce edema particularly in patients with lymphoma.
- When the tumor is chemosensitive, chemotherapy-naïve patients may benefit from such treatment.
- When the tumor is not chemosensitive and the patient has an adequately long prognosis, the preferred treatment is radiation therapy.

## Table 54. Management of Anorexia and Cachexia[85,86]

**Step 1 Discuss management strategy with the patient and family**

- Improve the patient's and family's understanding of anorexia and cachexia and the limitations of treatment.
- Explain that forcing patients to eat has no positive effect on well-being or survival.
- Explain that parenteral nutrition is associated with morbidity and lack of benefit and is not appropriate for most patients with cancer. Parenteral nutrition has serious side effects in 15% of patients, and the financial cost is very high.
- Encourage favorite foods for comfort and enjoyment; nutritional value is of limited importance.
- Develop realistic treatment goals that meet the patient's and family's needs.

**Step 2 Remove underlying cause**

Remove the underlying cause, if possible, and treat exacerbating conditions such as constipation, oral candida, nausea, pain, and depression.

**Step 3 Attempt to improve the patient's quality of life**

- Relieve nausea with pharmacologic therapy. (See Tables 69–71, pages, 118-123.)
- Attempt to improve appetite if severe anorexia is a major symptom and a source of distress for the patient.
  - Gastrointestinal motility agents (e.g., metoclopramide, or domperidone*)
  - Corticosteroids (e.g., dexamethasone 4–10 mg bid PO or SC). A trial of steroids is recommended to improve appetite. If successful, continue and taper slowly during the next few weeks. Taper more rapidly if trial unsuccessful. Prolonged use should be avoided. Improvement in appetite is temporary with no associated weight gain. Other benefits may include an improved sense of well-being and control of nausea. Monitor for side effects (e.g., mania) and complications.
  - Progestational agents (e.g., megestrol acetate). Start at 160 mg/d and increase up to 480 mg/d depending on results. An initial 2–4 week trial is advisable. Appetite stimulation lasts longer than with steroids. Avoid in presence of high risk for thromboembolic episodes.
  - Dronabinol (Marinol) has been proven effective in HIV patients. Start with 2.5 mg PO bid and titrate up to 20 mg/d, watching for mental disturbances and prohibitive cost.
  - Testosterone (topical, transdermal, or IM) or other androgens can be effective if hypogonadism is present.

*Not presently available in the United States.

## Table 55. Medical Management of Bowel Obstruction[85,86]

| Symptom | Drug | Dose | Comment |
|---|---|---|---|
| **Pain** | Morphine or hydromorphone | Titrate to relief PO, SL, SC, or IV (remember morphine SC dose = 1/3 PO dose and hydromorphone SC dose = 1/5 PO dose) | For cramping pain (colic), may need high dosage or addition of glycopyrrolate 0.8–2.0 mg/d SC or hyoscyamine (Levsin SL) 0.125 mg SL q 4–8 hours. If pain unrelieved, consider celiac plexus block. |
| **Nausea** | Haloperidol (Haldol) | 5–15 mg/d SC, PO, or IV | Mix in 5% dextrose for SC infusion. |
| | Metoclopramide (Reglan) | 60–240 mg/d SC, PO, or IV | May cause colic if opioid dose low. Better in patients with subtotal obstruction. |
| | Hydroxyzine (Vistaril) | 100–200 mg/d SC, PO, or IV | Add to haloperidol if necessary. |
| | Chlorpromazine (Thorazine) | 25–100 mg/tid PO, PR, or IV | Suppositories useful if SC infusion of above agents is unavailable. Sedating. |
| **Persistent Vomiting of Secretions (despite above measures)** | Octreotide (Sandostatin) | 0.1–0.6 mg/d by continuous SC infusion or bolus bid–tid | Expensive; reduces gut secretions[87] |
| **Constipation (in subtotal obstruction)** | Docusate | 100 mg PO bid–q 4 hours | Less likely to cause colic than stimulant laxatives. |
| | Dexamethasone | 4 mg PO or SC bid-qid | May relieve obstruction caused by bowel wall edema, but discontinued if ineffective in 5 days. |

## Table 56. Delirium—Assessment, Family Education, and General Treatment[85,86]

Delirium is characterized by the following *DSM-IV* criteria[90]:

- Clouding of consciousness or reduced ability to focus, sustain, or shift attention
- Perceptual disturbance, disorientation, or memory deficit that is not better accounted for by an established dementia
- Acute onset (hours to days) and a fluctuating course
- General evidence from the history and physical or laboratory findings of a medical condition related to the disturbance

**Step 1: Assessment**

- Maintain a high index of suspicion for delirium. It can be life threatening; proper assessment is essential.
- Use a screening tool to assess cognition, even in patients who do not appear confused. Do not rely solely on orientation questions.
- Ask specifically about hallucinations (usually visual and tactile) and paranoid ideation.
- Examine and look for signs of infection, opioid toxicity (myoclonus, hyperalgesia), dehydration, uremia, hepatic encephalopathy, etc.
- Order investigations when appropriate (e.g., complete blood cell count, electrolytes, calcium [with albumin], urea and creatinine, urinalysis, Chest x-ray, oxygen saturations).

**Step 2: Family and staff education**

- The treatment goal is comfort, not prolongation of life.
- Confusion and agitation are expressions of brain malfunction. Misinterpretation of symptoms as pain can result in excessive use of opioids, resulting in aggravation of the agitation.
- Most patients have limited or no recollection of their symptoms after the episode subsides.
- Hypoactive delirium can be misdiagnosed as depression and treated inappropriately with antidepressants.
- Delirium may be superimposed on pre-existing dementia unrecognized by family or health-care professionals.
- Urinary retention and constipation in cognitively impaired patients can be misdiagnosed as agitated delirium or "crescendo" pain.

**Step 3: Treatment of the underlying cause, if appropriate**

- **Opioid toxicity:** Change to another opioid, and reduce the dose if possible.
- **Sepsis:** Start antibiotics if appropriate, considering the goals of care.

*continued*

## Table 56: Delirium—Assessment, Family Education, and General Treatment[85,86] *(continued)*

**Step 3: Treatment of the underlying cause, if appropriate** *(continued)*

- **Drugs:** Stop, wean, or decrease possible offending drugs (e.g., tricyclic antidepressants, benzodiazepines). Nonsteroidal antiinflammatory drugs or angiotensin-converting enzyme inhibitors can cause renal failure leading to uremia or opioid metabolite accumulation.
- **Dehydration:** Start intravenous infusion or hypodermoclysis with saline (if the site leaks or swelling is uncomfortable, give 150 U hyaluronidase into the subcutaneous site before infusion; usually unnecessary); reassess daily. Do not give hyaluronidase intravenously.
- **Hypercalcemia:** See Table 53, page 98, "Management of Emergent Condition."
- **Hypoxia:** Treat underlying cause if possible and administer oxygen.
- **Urosepsis:** If possible, remove indwelling urinary catheter and treat infection with appropriate antibiotics.

**Step 4: Treatment of agitation/hallucinations**

See Table 57, page 106.

## Table 57. Treatment of Moderate to Severe Agitated Delirium*

**Moderate Delirium**

- Haloperidol (Haldol) 1–2 mg PO or SC hourly as needed to calm a crisis, then q 6–12 hours PO or by infusion
- If more sedation is needed, or for AIDS dementia complex, consider:

  – Thioridazine (Mellaril) 25–50 mg PO hourly until calm, then q 6–12 hours

  OR

  – Chlorpromazine (Thorazine) 25–50 mg PO, PR, or IV hourly until calm, then q 6–12 hours or by infusion

**Severe Agitated Delirium**

- Lorazepam (Ativan) 1–2 mg hourly, PO, SL, or IV + neuroleptic (as above)
- Midazolam (Versed) 0.4–4 mg/hour continuous SC (a mean dose of 2.9 mg/h [70 mg/d] was effective in 22 of 23 patients in one series)[91]
- Chlorpromazine (Thorazine) 100 mg q hour IV, PO, PR
- Some patients are helped by a combination of Haloperidol (Haldol) 5–20 mg/d and midazolam (Versed) 10–100 mg/d via continuous subcutaneous infusion.

**Rare Cases**

When none of the above methods work during the final hours of a patient's life, consider therapeutic sedation. (See Tables 92–93, pages 143 and 144.)

- Phenobarbital 130 mg SC hourly until calm and then by subcutaneous infusion (600–1,200 mg/d)[92]

  OR

- Thiopental (20–200 mg/h) or methohexital sodium (Brevital) continuous IV infusion titrated to unconsciousness[93,94]

*PO, orally; SC, subcutaneously; PR, per rectum; IV, intravenously.

## Table 58. Constipation: Causes, Symptoms, Treatments[85,86]

| Causes | Symptoms | Treatments |
| --- | --- | --- |
| • Malnutrition: autonomic neuropathy related to the anorexia/cachexia/asthenia syndrome of advanced cancer<br>• Drugs: opioids, anticholinergic drugs, diuretics, iron, etc.<br>• Poor fluid intake/dehydration<br>• Decreased mobility<br>• Abdominal tumors<br>• Hypokalemia, hypercalcemia | • Irregular bowel movements<br>• Diarrhea<br>• Nausea and vomiting<br>• Abdominal discomfort<br>• Bowel obstruction | • Digital rectal exam. Consistency of stool can guide treatment. When stool is hard, increase stool softeners (e.g., docusate). When stool is soft, try bisacodyl or senna.<br>• Encourage adequate fluid intake.<br>• Start laxatives simultaneously with initiation of opioid therapy.<br>• Start with a bowel stimulant and a stool softener (e.g., senna 1–2 tablets hs + docusate 100–240 mg bid PO). (Senna is available in rectal formulation if the patient is unable to swallow.)<br>• Titrate up to senna 2–4 tabs bid–qid + docusate 240 mg tid–qid, if needed.<br>• If no bowel movement within 3 days, administer a fleet enema or bisacodyl suppository rectally on day 3. If still no bowel movement, administer an oil retention enema followed by a soap suds enema several hours later (Caution: Do not use soap suds enema on debilitated, frail patients; use high phospho-soda enema [fleet].)<br>• If impaction in proximal colon, try magnesium citrate up to 250 mL PO.<br>• If rectum is empty on rectal exam, a plain abdominal X-ray may be useful. If bowel obstruction, treat appropriately. (See Table 55, page 103.)<br>• **If the above treatments are followed, manual disimpaction is seldom necessary.** If it must be done, premedicate with an opioid or midazolam. |

## Table 59. Cough: Causes and Treatments

| Causes | Treatments |
|---|---|
| Bronchitis or pneumonia | Antibiotic, oxygen, pulmonary toilet |
| Congestive heart failure | Diuretics, angiotensin-converting enzyme inhibitors, nitrates, inotropic agents |
| Pleural effusion | Diuresis or thoracentesis with/without pleurodesis |
| Aspiration | Thicken liquids and puree solids |
| Trachea-bronchial fistula | Esophageal stent |
| Allergic rhinitis, post-nasal drip | Antihistamine, possibly with<br>– decongestant<br>– steroid nasal spray |
| Lymphangitic spread of cancer into lungs | High-dose steroid |
| Angiotensin-converting enzyme inhibitors side effect | Discontinue medication |
| Secretion clearance problems | • Expectorant or nebulized saline (if strong cough)<br>• Anticholinergic<br>• See Tables 62 and 73, pages 112 and 125. |

If the above measures are not applicable or prove ineffective,

- Benzonatate (Tessalon) 100 mg PO q 4–8 hours
- Dextromethorphan 15–30 mg PO qid
- Increase opioid dose 25%–50% (or add codeine 15–30 mg PO q 4 hours)
- Lidocaine 5 ml of 2% solution per nebulizer q 4 hours
- If all else fails and cough is very distressing at the end of life, consider therapeutic sedation. See Tables 92–93, pages 143 and 144.

## Table 60. Diarrhea: Causes and Treatments

**Definition:** Diarrhea is defined as more than 3–4 loose stools per day.

### Causes

- Most common cause in cancer patients is laxative overdose.
- Other causes include bowel obstruction, fecal impaction, malabsorption, infectious agents, medications (e.g., antibiotics, antacids, iron), HIV disease (e.g., bacterial, protozoal, viral pathogens), radiotherapy, prior gastrointestinal surgery, hemorrhage, or concurrent medical illness.

### General Treatment

Directed at underlying causes and general supportive measures, including

- maintaining hydration (if appropriate)
- protecting the perianal area with products such as topical zinc oxide or cortisone preparations
- using antidiarrheal agents (See below.)

### Specific Treatment

- Treat enteric infections.
- Discontinue or adjust dose of laxatives.
- Radiation induced diarrhea: aspirin 325 mg q 4–6 hours; cholestyramine, 4 g tid
- Fat malabsorption: pancreatic enzyme replacement, 1–3 tablets with meals, 1 tablet with snacks
- Ileal resection: cholestyramine 4 g tid
- Carcinoid syndrome: cyproheptadine 4 mg tid–qid; octreotide 100–600 mcg/d in 2 divided doses given SC or IV
- Clostridium difficile colitis: metronidazole (Flagyl) or vancomycin orally
- Intestinal obstruction (See Table 55, page 103.)

### General Measures

- Opioids: codeine 10–60 mg q 4 hours, Loperamide 4 mg initial dose, then 2 mg after each loose stool up to 12–16 mg/d
- Diphenoxylate 10 mg initial dose, then 5 mg q 6 hours prn. High doses can cause anticholinergic side effects.
- Bulk forming agents: psyllium 1–2 teaspoons bid–tid; methylcellulose 1 tablespoon qd–tid (Use with care—may cause impaction.)

## Table 61. Dysphagia: Causes and Treatments

| Condition | Treatments |
|---|---|
| Dry mouth caused by radiation | • Pilocarpine 5–10 mg tid (watch for troublesome respiratory secretions or diarrhea)[95]<br>• Saliva substitute every 1–2 hours or chewing gum<br>• Pilocarpine + saliva substitute |
| Dryness caused by drugs | • Reduce dosage if possible.<br>• Change the medication (e.g., use metoclopramide [Reglan] or haloperidol [Haldol] instead of prochlorperazine [Compazine] or chlorpromazine [Thorazine]; use SSRI or trazodone [Desyrel] instead of amitriptyline [Elavil]).<br>• Apply fluoride to prevent dental damage. |
| Oral candidiasis | • Nystatin suspension, 5 mL swish and swallow qid<br>• Clotrimazole (Mycelex) 10 mg troches, one troche dissolved in mouth five times daily. (Patient compliance may be a problem when dry mouth is also present.)<br>• Ketoconazole (Nizoral), 200 mg 1–2 tablets daily for 10–14 days<br>• Fluconazole (Diflucan) 100 mg 1–2 times daily for 5–14 days |
| Bacterial infection | • The most common cause is periodontal disease. Consider adequate oral hygiene and an antibiotic or chlorhexidine (Peridex) oral rinse. |
| Viral infection | • Acyclovir (Zovirax) 400 mg five times daily for 7–10 days<br>• Famciclovir (Famvir) 500 mg PO bid for 7 days<br>• Valacyclovir (Valtrex) 500 mg PO bid for 3–10 days |
| Reflux esophagitis | • Omeprazole (Prilosec) 20 mg daily or other proton pump inhibitor<br>• Famotidine (Pepcid) 20 mg every 12 hours, or other $H_2$ blocking agent<br>• Place patient in more upright position by putting bricks under the head of the bed |

*continued*

**Table 61. Dysphagia: Causes and Treatments** *(continued)*

| Condition | Treatments |
|---|---|
| Mucosal damage from other causes such as aphthous ulcers[96] | • Chlorhexidine (Peridex) or oral lavage with 1 teaspoon of sodium bicarbonate (baking soda) to 1 quart of water<br>• Combination mouthwash utilizing 2–3 of the following:<br>– diphenhydramine (Benadryl)<br>– viscous xylocaine<br>– Maalox or kaopectate<br>– nystatin<br>– tetracycline<br>– hydrocortisone<br>• Xylocaine (Lidocaine) viscous 2%, 2–5 mL every 4–8 hours (can be diluted or flavored if desired). Can cause aspiration if used before meals.<br>• Sucralfate (Carafate) suspension 5 mL swish and swallow 3–4 times daily<br>• Parenteral opioids<br>• Thalidomide 200 mg daily (known to cause malformations in infants born to women taking this drug) |
| Dryness caused by systemic dehydration | • Increase liquid intake by mouth if possible. Try frozen juice or flavored ices.<br>• Ice chips, atomizer, and sips of water. (As death approaches, encouraging family members to keep the patient's mouth moist with a few drops of water from a syringe or a moist sponge stick involves them in the patient's care and relieves dry mouth.)[97]<br>• In selected patients, consider gentle (~1 L/d) rehydration with D5 1/2 normal saline by IV or SC infusion; if the site leaks or swelling is uncomfortable, put 150 U hyaluronidase (Wydase) into the SC site before infusion; usually unnecessary.[98] |

## Table 62. Dyspnea: Specific Causes and Treatments

| | |
|---|---|
| **B** | **Bronchospasm.** If present, consider nebulized albuterol or inhalers and/or oral steroids; if not present, consider lowering doses of theophylline and adrenergic agents to reduce any tremor and anxiety, which often exacerbate dyspnea. |
| **R** | **Rales.** If volume overload is present, reduce artificial feeding or stop intravenous fluids. Diuretics are occasionally needed. If pneumonia seems likely, decide whether an antibiotic will rehabilitate the patient or just prolong the dying process. Patient and family participation in this decision is essential. |
| **E** | **Effusions.** Thoracentesis can be effective; if the effusion recurs and the patient is ambulatory, consider chest tube pleurodesis or indwelling drainage catheter. If the patient is close to death, palliate the dyspnea with opioids and benzodiazepines. |
| **A** | **Airway obstruction.** Make sure tracheostomy appliances are cleaned regularly. If aspiration of food is likely, purée solids and thicken liquids with cornstarch or "Thick-it." Instruct the family on positioning the patient during feeding and suctioning if necessary. |
| **T** | **Thick secretions.** If the cough reflex is still strong, loosen secretions with nebulized saline and an expectorant as needed. If the cough is weak, dry secretions with hyoscyamine (Levsin) 0.125 mg orally or sublingual q 8 hours or Transderm Scop 1–3 patches every 3 days, or add glycopyrrolate 0.8–2.0 mg/d to a subcutaneous infusion or by subcutaneous or intravenous bolus 0.4 mg q 3 hours prn. These drugs also reduce the so-called "death rattle." (Also see Tables 59 and 73, pages 108 and 125.) |
| **H** | **Hemoglobin low.** A blood transfusion may improve energy and reduce dyspnea for a few weeks.[99] Although costly, consider erythropoietin (Procrit, Epogen) for patients likely to improve to a higher functional level. More often, hemorrhage or marrow failure are part of the dying process and are best palliated with opioids, benzodiazepines, and other symptomatic treatments. |
| **A** | **Anxiety.** The following can be extremely effective: sitting upright, using a bedside fan, listening to calming music, and practicing relaxation techniques, as well as skillful counseling and the presence of a calming physician. Dyspnea exacerbates normal fears and anxiety, so treat it first with a short-acting opioid (e.g., morphine 2.5–20 mg q 1 hour prn), then try a short-acting benzodiazepine if needed (lorazepam 0.5–2 mg PO/PR/IV, or alprazolam 0.25–1 mg PO q 3–8 hours prn). If the patient is already being treated with opioids, titrate the opioid dose by 25%–50% above the existing dose. If the opioid dose is limited by drowsiness, reduce the benzodiazepine and increase the opioid. |
| **I** | **Interpersonal issues.** Social and financial problems contribute to dyspnea. Counseling with social workers and other members of the interdisciplinary team may bring relief. When family relationships exacerbate the problem, a few days in an inpatient unit may help relieve the patient's symptoms. |
| **R** | **Religious concerns.** Although faith or an experience of the transcendent can bring profound comfort, some beliefs, such as "God is punishing me" or "God will heal me if I have enough faith," can precipitate dyspnea and/or exacerbate its symptoms. Take time to listen with full attention and presence. Help patients explore ways to reconnect with God, the cosmos, or the deepest parts of the self. Coordinate treatment with the patient's spiritual adviser, chaplain, counselor, other healthcare professionals, and family members. |

## Table 63. General Measures for Treating Dyspnea

**General treatment measures for dyspnea include the following:**

- Reduce the need for exertion and arrange for readily available help.
- Reposition, usually to a more upright position or with the compromised lung down.
- Improve air circulation.
  - Provide a draft—use fans, open windows.
  - Adjust humidity with humidifier or air conditioner.
- Address anxiety and provide reassurance.
  - Discuss need for companionship and spiritual support. Isolation and spiritual concerns can exacerbate symptoms.
  - Discuss the meaning of symptoms and other patient/family concerns.
  - Anticipate and rehearse with the patient/family their responses when symptoms worsen.
  - Identify situational components (i.e., What triggers the dyspnea attack?).
  - Teach behavioral interventions such as relaxation and hypnosis.
- Discuss any patient/family/staff concerns about using opioids to relieve dyspnea.

## Table 64. Opioid Therapy for Treating Dyspnea

**Mild Dyspnea in Patients Taking No Pain Medications**

Begin with low doses of an opioid such as hydrocodone or acetaminophen with codeine. (Children and the elderly may require lower doses, so break tablets in half or consider hydrocodone syrup [5 mg/5 mL] 1–3 mL q 4 hours with booster doses of the full 4-hour dose prn)

- Hydrocodone (Hycodan or Lortab) 5 mg tablet q 4 hours with a booster dose of 5 mg q 2 hours prn

OR

- Acetaminophen with codeine (Tylenol #3) 30 mg (1 tablet) q 4 hours with a booster dose of 30 mg q 2 hours prn

**Severe Dyspnea or Dyspnea Being Treated With Opioids Such as Codeine, Hydrocodone, or Propoxyphene**

Consider switching to a more potent oral opioid such as

- Oxycodone 3–10 mg q 4 hours prn
- Morphine syrup 3–10 mg q 4 hours prn
- Hydromorphone (Dilaudid) tablets 0.5–2 mg q 4 hours prn

**Severe Dyspnea in Patients Already Being Treated with Opioids Such as Oxycodone, Morphine, or Hydromorphone, and those with High Levels of Anxiety**

Consider increasing the above doses by up to 50% q 4–12 hours until the patient experiences relief. Treatment in an inpatient hospice/palliative care setting may be appropriate because close monitoring is essential. In addition, subcutaneous administration of escalating doses of opioids and midazolam (Versed) may be required. The entire interdisciplinary team should be involved in interventions for severe dyspnea.

**Use of Oxygen**

Opioids are the first-choice treatment agents for most nonspecific dyspnea associated with terminal illness. Because opioids are so effective, supplemental oxygen often is unnecessary in palliative care. When oxygen is required to help relieve severe dyspnea, nasal prongs may be all that is needed because opioids tend to reduce the patient's oxygen requirements. If possible, oxygen masks should be avoided because they isolate the patient and can be frightening.

## Table 65. Managing Refractory Dyspnea

- Look for treatable causes (e.g., airway obstruction, bronchospasm, pulmonary edema).
- Consider escalating the opioid dose. (See Table 64, page 114.)
- Consider a trial of dexamethasone 2–4 mg bid, PO or SC.
- Consider an opioid infusion IV or SC, with boluses for breakthrough dyspnea.
- Consider nebulized morphine or hydromorphone (use 5%–15% of the daily dose q 4 hours prn).
- Consider adding midazolam 2–20 mg/d to the opioid infusion.

## Table 66. Proposed Criteria for Fatigue in Cancer and Other Progressive Illnesses[102]

Fatigue is an abnormal condition persisting for at least 2 weeks.

- Major Characteristics
  - sensation of fatigue, diminished energy, increased need to rest not proportional to activity
  - distressing or associated with diminished capacity to perform
  - causally related to the disease or a treatment
  - no evidence of being related to a comorbid psychiatric disorder
- Patient may use other descriptors
  - diminished motivation, volition, mental acuity, interest in activities, or ability to attend to activities
  - feelings of exhaustion, apathy, or lassitude
  - sense of generalized weakness, without true loss of motor function
  - sense of sleepiness, increased need for daytime sleep, insomnia, or nonrestorative sleep
  - mood disturbances described as irritability or sadness

Adapted from Portenoy RK, Miaskowski C. Assessment and management of cancer-related fatigue. In: Berger A, Portenoy RK, Weissman DE, eds. *Principles and Practice of Supportive Oncology.* Philadelphia: Lippincott-Raven Publishers. 1998: 109–118.

## Table 67. Management of Fatigue

**Pharmacological**

- Pharmacological management is directed at the cause of the symptom.
- A trial of prednisone and/or methylphenidate may be helpful.
- A blood transfusion or a trial of erythropoietin to stimulate red blood cell production may be appropriate and may partially relieve fatigue.
- Fatigue associated with simple dehydration may be corrected with a short course of hypodermoclysis or intravenous fluids.
- Testosterone injections or gel may be helpful for men with HIV.

**Nonpharmacological**

- Tailor treatments to the patient's prognosis, and involve members of an interdisciplinary team.
- Arrange for a physical therapy consult and exercise recommendations to promote the patient's and family's sense of independence and control while investigating etiology.
- Ask patient to keep a diary of energy levels during the day and sleep patterns during the day and night.
- Arrange for frequent, brief visits from the healthcare team to provide emotional support and reassurance.
- Encourage activities such as reading, listening to music, and engaging in a hobby to retain a sense of creativity and usefulness.
- Rearrange the patient's room to remove impediments to activity.

## Table 68. Hiccups: Causes and Treatments

| Causes | Treatments |
|---|---|
| Gastric distension | • Reduce tube feeding<br>• Metoclopramide |
| Esophageal reflux | $H_2$ blocker (e.g., ranitidine) or proton pump[103] inhibitor (e.g., lansoprazole) |
| Anxiety | Calm environment |
| Drug induced (benzodiazepines, corticosteroids, barbiturates) | Stop, wean, or decrease the drug |
| Electrolyte imbalance | Supplement deficiency |
| Nonpharmacologic treatments | • Hold breath, drink water slowly, breathe into a paper bag<br>• Swallow granulated sugar or dry bread<br>• Stimulate palate with cotton swab or rubber catheter<br>• Carotid sinus massage or Valsalva maneuver |
| Pharmacologic treatments | • Baclofen 10–20 mg PO tid<br>• Chlorpromazine 25–50 mg PO, IV, IM qd–qid<br>• Haloperidol 1–4 mg PO or SC tid<br>• Metoclopramide 10–20 mg PO or SC qid<br>• Nifedipine 10–20 mg PO q 8 hours<br>• Valproate 250–500 mg PO tid<br>• Phenytoin 200 mg IV or 300–400 PO qd<br>• Midazolam 10–60 mg/d by SC infusion |

## Table 69. Nausea: Causes and Treatments

| Specific Cause | Look for | Consider |
|---|---|---|
| **Cortical** | | |
| Tumor in central nervous system or meninges | Neurologic signs or mental status problems | • Dexamethasone 4–8 mg PO/SC q 4–8 hours<br>• Consider radiation therapy for new metastases |
| Increased intracranial pressure | Projectile vomiting, headache | • Dexamethasone 4–8 mg PO/SC q 4–8 hours |
| Anxiety and other conditioned responses | Anticipatory nausea, predictable vomiting | • Counseling<br>• Benzodiazepines (e.g., lorazepam 0.5–1.5 mg PO q 4–8 hours) |
| Uncontrolled pain | Pain and nausea | • Opiates, other pain medications, adjuvants |
| **Vestibular/Middle Ear** | | |
| Vestibular disease | Vertigo or vomiting after head motion | • Meclizine 25 mg PO tid<br>• Ear, nose, throat consult |
| Middle ear infections | Ear pain or bulging tympanic membrane | • Antibiotic and/or decongestant as appropriate |
| Motion sickness | Travel-related nausea | • Transderm Scop<br>• Dimenhydrinate 50 mg PO tid PRN |
| **Chemoreceptor Trigger Zone**<br>The most common causes of nausea are mediated by this area in the brain, which senses changes in the blood. | | |
| Drugs (e.g., opiates, digoxin, chemotherapy, carbamazepine, antibiotics, theophylline) | Nausea worse after drug started, exacerbated by increased dose | • Decrease drug dose or discontinue drug if possible |
| Metabolic (e.g., renal or liver failure or tumor products) | Increased blood urea nitrogen, creatinine, bilirubin | • Haloperidol PO or SC or ondansetron (Zofran) PO or SC |
| Hyponatremia | Confusion, low sodium | • Salt tablets<br>• Demeclocycline |
| Hypercalcemia | Somnolence, delirium, high calcium | • Hydration and pamidronate 60–90 mg IV |

*continued*

**Table 69. Nausea: Causes and Treatments** *(continued)*

| Specific Cause | Look for | Consider |
|---|---|---|
| **Gastrointestinal Tract** | | |
| Irritation by drugs | Use of nonsteroidal antiinflammatory drugs, iron, alcohol, antibiotics | • Stop drug, if possible, proton pump inhibitor, add misoprostol or H2 blocker, |
| Tumor infiltration, radiation therapy to the gastrointestinal tract, or infection | Candida esophagitis, colitis, history of x-ray therapy | • Haloperidol SC/PO, possibly with hydroxyzine SC/PO, treat infection<br>• Transderm Scop |
| Constipation or impaction | • Abdominal distension<br>• Long time since last bowel movement | • Laxative, manual disimpaction prn, enema |
| Obstruction by tumor or poor motility | • Constipation unrelieved by treatment<br>• Response to motility agent | • Metoclopramide (Reglan) |
| Tube feedings | Abdominal distension, diarrhea | • Reduce feeding volume |
| Gag reflex from feeding tube | Vomiting after nasogastric insertion | • Remove it |
| Nasopharyngeal bleeding | • Hemoptysis, epistaxis<br>• Blood visible in pharynx | • Packing, vitamin K if appropriate, sedation |
| Thick secretions | Cough-induced vomiting | • Nebulized saline expectorant if good cough reflex; anticholinergic if poor cough reflex |

## Table 70. Antiemetic Guide: Pharmacologic Management

| Class of Drug | Initial Dose PO | Initial Dose Parenteral | Comments |
|---|---|---|---|
| **Prokinetic Agents** | | | |
| Metoclopramide (Reglan) | 5-15 mg before meals and at bedtime. For children, 0.5mg/kg/ dose to max of 15mg/dose | SC/IV = PO | • For nausea and gastric stasis from various causes<br>• May cause dystonia, which is reversible with diphenhydramine 1.0 mg/kg<br>• Antiemetic dose is greater than pro-kinetic dose of 0.1–0.2 mg/kg/dose<br>• Well tolerated SC |
| **Antihistamines** | | | |
| Diphenhydramine (Benadryl) | 1 mg/kg/dose PO q 4 hours to a max of 100 mg/dose | SC/IV = PO | • Sedating<br>• Can cause confusion in elderly patients |
| Hydroxyzine (Atarax) | 0.5–1.0 mg/kg/ dose q 4 hours to a max of 600 mg/d | SC/IV = PO | • More sedating at higher doses<br>• Skin irritation when given SC |
| Promethazine (Phenergan) | 0.25–1 mg/kg q 4 hours | IV = PO = PR | • Can cause dystonia (phenothiazine derivative) |
| **Neuroleptics**<br>• Can cause dystonia, reversible with diphenhydramine 1 mg/kg or benztropine (Cogentin) 0.02–0.05 mg/kg/dose to max of 4 mg IV<br>• IV can cause postural hypotension<br>• Give IV slowly | | | |
| Haloperidol (Haldol) | 0.5–5 mg/dose q 8 hours up to 30 mg/d; for children 0.01–0.05 mg/kg/dose up to q 8 hours | SC/IV = 1/2 PO | • Use care: only some preparations can be given IV.<br>• Use D5W to dilute.<br>• Well tolerated SC. |
| Chlorpromazine (Thorazine) | 0.5 to 1.0 mg/kg q 8 hours | IV = PO | • More sedating<br>• Irritating to tissue when given SC |

*continued*

## Table 70. Antiemetic Guide: Pharmacologic Management *(continued)*

| Class of Drug | Initial Dose PO | Initial Dose Parenteral | Comments |
|---|---|---|---|
| **Neuroleptics** *(continued)* | | | |
| Prochlorperazine (Compazine) | 0.15 mg/kg/dose q 4 hours to a max of 10 mg/dose | IV = PO = PR | • Irritating to tissues when given SC |
| **Serotonin 5HT3 receptor antagonists:** | | | |
| Ondansetron (Zofran) | 0.15 mg/kg/dose q 6 hours to max of 32 mg/d | IV = PO | • Particularly helpful in chemotherapy-induced nausea and vomiting, costly |
| Granisetron (Kytril) | 0.04 mg/kg q 8 hours to max of 2 mg/d | 0.01–0.02 mg/kg | • same as above<br>• not approved in children |
| **Benzodiazepines** | | | |
| Diazepam (Valium, Diastat) | 0.05–0.2 mg/kg/dose q 6 hours | <5 years: max = 5 mg/dose; > 5 years: max = 10 mg/dose | • Helpful for anticipatory nausea and vomiting<br>• Diazepam stings IV: dilute and use large vein if possible |
| Lorazepam (Ativan) | 0.03–0.05 mg/kg/dose q 6 hours to max of 4 mg/dose | IV = PO/SL | |
| **Corticosteroids** | | | |
| Dexamethasone (Decadron) | 6–10 mg loading dose, then 2–4 mg bid–qid for maintenance<br>if <10 kg, 1 mg/kg loading + 0.1 mg/kg maintenance | SC/IV = PO | • Helpful with hepatic capsular distension, anorexia, increased intracranial pressure<br>• Well tolerated SC<br>• Beware of long-term side effects<br>• Mood swings |
| Prednisone | 1.5 mg dexamethasone = 10 mg prednisone | N/A | |

*continued*

## Table 70. Antiemetic Guide: Pharmacologic Management *(continued)*

| | Initial Dose | | |
|---|---|---|---|
| **Class of Drug** | **PO** | **Parenteral** | **Comments** |
| **Cannabinoids** | | | |
| Dronabinol (Marinol) | 2.5 mg bid (adult) to max of 20 mg/d | N/A | • Can cause dysphoria, drowsiness, or hallucinations |
| **Other Anticholinergics** | | | |
| Scopolamine | Transdermal preparation—1.5 mg patch delivers 0.5 mg over 3 days | 0.006 mg/kg/dose q 6 hours IV/SC | • Helpful with motion/movement-related nausea and vomiting<br>• Well tolerated by SC tissues<br>• Often causes dry mouth, blurred vision, and sometimes confusion |

*Notes:*

N/A Not available; Max = maximum dose

Doses are simply guidelines for initial dosing, as are the intervals given as the shortest time between initial dosing. Dose and interval can be titrated to relief or side effect. May be given on prn or scheduled basis.

## Table 71. Managing Refractory Nausea

- Look for reversible causes (e.g., drug reaction, constipation, anxiety).
- Look for bowel obstruction and consider surgery if appropriate; see Table 55, page 103.
  - Consider an IV or SC infusion of an opioid, haloperidol (2–10 mg/d), and an anticholinergic (e.g., glycopyrrolate 0.6–2.0 mg/d).
  - Consider a trial of dexamethasone 4–8 mg/d.
  - Consider octreotide 100–300 mcg/d by IV or SC via bid bolus or continuous infusion.
- Consider adding a second or third potent antiemetic (metoclopramide, hydroxyzine, or chlorpromazine) and escalating the dose.
- Consider changing to an IV or SC infusion.
- Consider adding dexamethasone 2–8 mg bid.

## Table 72. Pruritus: Assessment and Management

| Cause | Treatment |
|---|---|
| • Drug reactions | Stop the drug. |
| • Drug-induced cholestasis<br>– estrogens<br>– androgens<br>– steroids<br>– phenothiazine<br>– antibiotics | Stop the drug, if possible. |
| • Malignant cholestasis | Biliary stent<br>Cholestyramine 4 g PO tid<br>Ondansetron<br>Phototherapy<br>Corticosteroid |
| • Infections of the skin<br>– scabies<br>– Candida | Treat infection |
| • Dry scaly skin (ichthyosis) | Moisturizing lotions and bath oils |
| • Polycythemia | Cimetidine $H_2$ blockade |
| • Intrathecal morphine | Naloxone |
| • Nonspecific pruritus<br>– topical therapy | • **Cool the skin**<br>– air conditioning/fan<br>– alcohol in bath<br>– menthol/camphor creams<br>– benzocaine spray<br>– topical steroid<br>• **EMLA cream**<br>• **Capsaicin cream or TENS** |
| – systemic therapy | • **Antihistamines** $H_1$ Blockade<br>– Hydroxyzine 10–25 mg PO/SC q 4–12 hours<br>– Cyproheptadine 4 mg PO q 8–12 hours<br>– Chlorpromazine 25–50 mg PO/IV q 6 hours<br>• **Anxiolytics**<br>– Hydroxyzine 10–50 mg PO/SC q 4–12 hours<br>– Diazepam 2–10 mg PO tid<br>– Doxepin 25–75 mg PO q hs<br>• **Corticosteroid**<br>Dexamethasone 2–8 mg PO or SC bid |
| • Other skin diseases | Dermatology consult |

## Table 73. Respiratory Secretions: Assessment and Management

| Symptom | Treatment |
|---|---|
| Aspiration of food or fluids | Feed upright; thicken liquids |
| Overhydration | Decrease IV fluids or tube feedings |
| Pneumonia or bronchitis | Antibiotics |
| Pulmonary edema | Diuretic |
| Tenacious secretions and strong cough | Nebulized saline tid (See Tables 59 and 62, pages 108 and 112.) |
| Too weak to cough | Hyoscyamine 0.125 mg SL or PO<br>OR<br>Glycopyrrolate 0.2–0.6 mg PO or SC tid |

## Table 74. Refractory Pain and Other Symptoms: Assessment and Management

1. Involve the entire interdisciplinary team in assessing and relieving physical, psychological, social, and spiritual distress. See *Unipac Three: Assessing and Treating Pain in the Terminally Ill.*
2. Obtain a consultation from experts in hospice and palliative medicine. See www.abhpm.org for a regional list of physicians certified by the American Board of Hospice and Palliative Medicine.
3. Consider an inpatient re-evaluation, especially in a hospice or palliative care inpatient unit.
4. Consider the use of sedation:
   - Consider the ethical implications. (See Table 91, page 142.)
   - Discuss available options and the goals of treatment with the interdisciplinary team and the patient and family.
   - Follow the process and principles of sedation. (See Tables 92–93, pages, 143 and 144.)
     - Partial or temporary sedation may be enough, perhaps with a benzodiazepine.
     - In extreme cases phenobarbital boluses or a thiopental infusion may be needed.
     - See *Unipac Six: Ethical and Legal Decision Making* for more information.[6]

# 5. Communication and the Physician's Role on an Interdisciplinary Team

## Communication

**Tables 75-79**, pages 128–131, outline effective strategies for communicating with patients and their families.

- **Table 75**, page 128, techniques to use in talking with patients
- **Table 76**, page 129, patients' preferences when physicians communicate bad news
- **Table 77**, page 129, a six-step protocol for communicating bad news
- **Table 78**, page 130, counseling techniques for use during family conferences
- **Table 79**, page 131, strategies to encourage family and patient communication about dying.

## The Interdisciplinary Team

**Table 80**, page 132, lists skills of effective team leaders.

## Managing Stress Experienced by Physicians

**Table 81**, page 132, lists signs and symptoms of stress overload in physicians, and **Table 82**, page 133, lists stress management strategies.

## Table 75. Techniques for Effective Communication with Patients

**Open-ended Questions**

Open-ended questions encourage patients to describe their symptoms more fully and to say more about what they are thinking and feeling. Examples: "What else can you tell me about where the pain is and how it feels?" "Can you tell me more about how you are feeling today?" "Can you tell me something about how your family is coping?"

**Minimal Leads and Accurate Verbal Following**

Minimal verbal leads indicate interest and encourage patients to continue talking (e.g., "uh-huh," "umm," "hmm," "ah").

**Repetition**

Repetition encourages patients to keep talking and enhances their sense of being heard. Example: Patient: "The pills I take make me feel nervous." Physician: "The pills make you feel nervous."

**Paraphrasing**

Paraphrasing involves repeating the patient's own words to ensure the message is understood. Examples: "Your medication wasn't delivered until 9 pm; when you took the pills, they kept you up all night." Or, "When you think about dying, you worry about uncontrollable pain."

**Clarifying Responses**

Clarifying responses help physicians understand the facts and the patient's feelings and attitudes. Examples: "Is it possible that you feel...?" "Can you give me an example of what you are talking about?" You say you are feeling good most of the time; what is going on when you are not feeling good?"

**Confrontation and Honest Labeling**

This is a technique for gently exploring uncomfortable subjects, such as distortions of reality or differences between words and actions. Example: "When you talk about your wife, you say that you understand why she doesn't visit you more often, but I see tears in your eyes. Can you tell me more about how you feel when she doesn't visit?"

**Integrating and Summarizing**

These techniques help ensure the patient's main concerns are understood. Example: "Let me see if I understand what you have told me. When the pain returned, you thought it meant you were going to die soon, which made you feel frightened and alone and you thought about ending your life. However, if the pain can be controlled and people come to visit you, you'd rather live a little longer because you have some important things you'd like to do before you die."

## Table 76. Patients' Preferences When Physicians Communicate Bad News[104]

| |
|---|
| • Direct, empathetic communication |
| • Information about diagnosis, which provides a label for their condition |
| • Information about prognosis and how the illness is likely to affect their quality of life |
| • Inclusion of a family member or trusted friend in the discussion |
| • Encouragement to ask questions |
| • Information that is neither overly optimistic nor overly pessimistic |
| • Practical information about what to do and how to obtain additional information |

## Table 77. A Six-Step Protocol for Communicating Bad News[105]

| |
|---|
| 1. Arrange the physical context and the emotional atmosphere. |
| 2. Find out how much the patient knows. |
| 3. Find out how much the patient wants to know. |
| 4. Share information (align and educate). |
| 5. Respond to the patient's feelings. |
| 6. Make a plan and follow through. |

## Table 78. Counseling Techniques for Use During Family Conferences

- Use listening techniques and nonverbal behaviors that communicate empathy and interest, encourage patients and family members to talk, indicate the physician is listening, and enhance the patient's and family's sense of being heard.
- Demystify and correct misconceptions, such as "using morphine causes addiction," or "when artificial nutrition is withheld, terminally ill patients suffer and their lives are shortened." (See *UNIPAC Three: Assessment and Treatment of Pain in the Terminally Ill*[3], *UNIPAC Four: Management of Selected, Non-pain Symptoms in the Terminally Ill*[4], and *UNIPAC Six: Ethical and Legal Decision Making When Caring for the Terminally Ill.*)
- Acknowledge the fear, grief, and guilt experienced by families who care for terminally ill patients (e.g., "If only I had fed him more, he wouldn't be so thin," and "If only I had taken her to a different doctor, she wouldn't be dying now").
- Exhibit equal loyalty to all members of the family, and refrain from taking sides with one or more family members.
- Help patients and family members identify their strengths and set realistic short-term goals.
- Use reframing to help patients and families recognize other perspectives. (See *UNIPAC Two: Alleviating Psychological and Spiritual Pain in the Terminally Ill.*[2])
- Help patients and families make sense of what is happening to them by engaging in an ongoing search for meaning. (See *UNIPAC Two: Alleviating Psychological and Spiritual Pain in the Terminally Ill.*[2])

## Table 79. Strategies to Encourage Family and Patient Communication About Dying

**Normalize Concerns**

Acknowledge the difficulty of talking about a serious illness.

**Assess Concerns**

- What are some of your concerns about sharing this information with the patient? (Will the family be forced to talk about death every moment of every day until the patient dies? Will the patient's life be miserable every moment of every day until life ends?)
- What is likely to happen if the information is not shared?
- What is the worst thing that is likely to happen if the information is not shared?
- What is likely to happen if the information is shared?
- What is the worst thing that is likely to happen if the information is shared?

**Educate**

- Provide information about the benefits of communicating with patients.
  - Studies indicate that most dying patients want more information about their diagnosis and prognosis than anyone realizes.
  - Most dying patients want to talk about death-related concerns.
  - Withholding information sets a pattern of deception that can destroy a patient's trust in the physician and members of the family.
  - Withholding information isolates patients and prevents them from planning for the future and making treatment-related decisions.
  - Ethically, physicians cannot refuse to share information with patients who ask for it.
  - Communication is part of a continuing dialogue about the patient's life (e.g., joys, struggles, successes, failures, and search for meaning).

## Table 80. Skills of Effective Team Leaders[106,107]

- Plan and facilitate meetings with clear objectives; stay on track.
- Encourage use of a problem-solving approach.
- Encourage comprehensive interventions that meet the needs of patients and families.
- Ensure effective coordination and communication.
- Share team decisions with necessary parties.
- Keep extraneous anecdotal information to a minimum.
- Help motivate other team members to the highest possible standards of care.
- Adapt leadership style to specific circumstances.
- Balance problem-solving and task-oriented behavior with nurturing and motivating.
- Encourage regularly scheduled self-evaluations to measure and improve the team's internal functioning and the effectiveness of its intervention to alleviate a patient's and family's suffering and improve their quality of life.

## Table 81. Signs and Symptoms of Stress Overload in Physicians[108,109]

- Tiredness out of proportion to the work that is being done
- Low morale
- Over-conscientiousness, loss of a sense of proportion, and preoccupation with patients
- Loss of sense of humor
- Conflicts with staff and scapegoating
- Avoidance of patients
- Difficulties at home
- Distancing, depersonalization, and intellectualization
- Anger, irritability, frustration
- Helplessness, inadequacy, and insecurity
- Depression, grief, and guilt
- Errors in judgment

**Table 82. Strategies for Managing Stress**[108,110,111]

- Develop a sense of competence.
- Develop practice patterns that enhance control and pleasure.
- Develop decision-making protocols.
- Develop collegial relationships with other professionals.
- Develop staffing policies that reduce stress.
- Develop a personal philosophy that provides a sense of meaning.
- Develop strategies that provide a sense of rejuvenation.
- Develop personal habits that increase the ability to cope with stress.
- Acknowledge life's imperfections.
- If necessary, find new professional opportunities.

# 6. Ethical and Legal Decision Making

## Ethical Principles

For information on the application of ethical principles to hospice/palliative care settings, see **Table 83**, page 136. For more information on ethical and legal decision making, see *UNIPAC Six: Ethical and Legal Desicion Making When Caring for the Terminally Ill.*[6]

## Competence and Decision-Making Capacity

**Table 84**, page 137, compares the patient's legal competence with the capacity to make healthcare decisions.

## Legal Myths

**Table 85**, page 138, describes current legal myths and realities.

**Table 86**, page 139, describes the status of previously identified legal myths.

## Advance Directives

**Table 87**, page 140, describes lists instructive and proxy advance directives.

See **Table 88**, page 140, for misconceptions about cardiopulmonary resuscitation and "Do not resuscitate" orders.

## Futility

See **Table 89**, page 141, for information on making decisions about futile treatment. See **Table 90**, pages 141–142, for data-gathering questions for physicians to use in connection with forgoing treatment.

## Sedation at the End of Life

**Table 91**, page 142, lists ethical considerations related to sedation at the end of life. **Table 92**, page 143, describes the process of sedation at the end of life. **Table 93**, page 144, lists the pharmacologic principles of sedation at the end of life.

## Table 83. Ethical Principles Applicable to Hospice/Palliative Care Settings

**Beneficence**

In hospice and other palliative care settings, the principle of beneficence implies positive acts such as treating pain and other symptoms effectively, and providing psychosocial and spiritual support.[112]

**Autonomy**

Patients with decision-making capacity are free to reject, without coercion or fear of retribution, any form of medical therapy, including life-prolonging or life-sustaining therapy.[113] A patient's right to refuse unwanted treatment, including nutrition and hydration, is absolute. In hospice and palliative care settings, the principle of autonomy includes the patient's right not only to refuse a particular course of treatment, but also to ask that the treatment be modified to meet other needs, such as the need for privacy, mental alertness, or care in a particular setting.[114]

**Nonmaleficence**

In hospice/palliative care settings, examples of possible violations of the principal of nonmaleficence include:[112]

- Insisting that patients confront the reality of their approaching death
- Destroying hope
- Providing unnecessary sedation
- Failing to stop treatments when the burden begins to exceed the benefit (e.g., continuing the provision of artificial nutrition when patients are actively dying, continuing to provide IV fluids for dyspneic patients with congestive heart failure).
- Failing to prescribe adequate doses of opioids or other medications to control pain and other distressing symptoms.

**Justice**

Justice may limit personal autonomy when patients' wishes conflict with the needs of society. Society cannot be expected to fund futile treatment (i.e., treatment that offers no reasonable hope of benefit).

**Virtue and Professional Integrity**

Virtues that define the character of a good physician include:[115]

- Fidelity to trust and promise—honoring the ineradicable trust of the patient-physician relationship
- Effacement of self-interest—protecting the patient from exploitation and refraining from using the patient as a means of advancing power, prestige, profit, or pleasure
- Compassion and caring—exhibiting concern, empathy, and consideration for the patient's plight
- Intellectual honesty—knowing when to say, "I do not know"
- Prudence—deliberating and discerning alternatives in situations of uncertainty and stress.

## Table 84. Legal Competence Versus Capacity to Make Healthcare Decisions

### Competence

The terms *competence* and *incompetence* refer to a person's ability to understand the nature and consequences of nonhealth-related decisions and are restricted to describing a person's legal status, as determined by a court of law. Competence is determined by a proper legal authority, usually a judge.[116]

### Capacity to Make Healthcare Decisions

*A patient is presumed to have decision-making capacity unless proven otherwise.*
Decision-making capacity refers to a person's ability to:[113,116]

Decision-specific

- understand and articulate relevant information and the implications of treatment choices
- reflect on information in accordance with personal values; draw and articulate conclusions
- make and articulate a choice to healthcare professionals.

Decision-making capacity is determined by a physician. It can be temporarily or permanently compromised by conditions such as delirium, dementia, metabolic imbalances, severe pain, life-threatening infection, high doses of drugs to control symptoms, advancing disease, and psychological factors such as the patient's denial of serious illness.[118]

In clinical settings, the physician should first assess the patient's mental status and look for treatable physical conditions that interfere with the ability to process information and draw conclusions.

When a patient's capacity fluctuates or is uncertain, there is no need to further clarify decision-making capacity if the physician, the patient/surrogate, and family members agree on treatment decisions. When disagreements about treatment occur, the best course of action is to wait, if possible, until the patient regains decision-making capacity. If a patient's lack of decision-making capacity is likely to continue indefinitely, the designated surrogate has the authority to make decisions in accordance with the following guidelines:[113]

- Follow the patient's advance directive.
- If no directive is available, apply the patient's preferences and values.
- If the patient's preferences and values are unknown, choose as a reasonable person would in the patient's circumstances.

Documentation in the patient's medical record is critical. It should include a description of how and with whom a decision of incapacity was reached.

## Table 85. Current Legal Myths and Realities [118]

| Current Myth | Reality |
|---|---|
| • Forgoing life-sustaining treatment for patients without decision-making capacity requires evidence that this was the patient's actual wish. | • Such treatment may be forgone if the patient's surrogate relates that this was the patient's actual wish, or, in most states, if it was the patient's probable wish. Only a few states require "clear and convincing" evidence of patient wishes. In a few states, it is even permissible to terminate life support with the surrogate's permission if the patient's wishes are not known, and when termination of treatment is in the patient's "best interests." |
| • Withholding or withdrawing of artificial fluids and nutrition from terminally ill or permanently unconscious patients is illegal. | • Like any other medical treatment, fluids and nutrition may be withheld or withdrawn if the patients refuses them or, in the case of an incapacitated patient, if the appropriate standards of surrogate decision-making are met. |
| • Risk management personnel must be consulted before life-sustaining medical treatment may be terminated. | • There is no legal or ethical requirement that a risk manager be consulted before making end-of-life decisions though some hospital policies may require it. |
| • Advance directive must comply with specific forms, are not transferable between states, and govern all future treatment decisions. Oral advance directives are unenforceable. | • Advance directives are the best indication of an incapacitated patient's wishes, and may guide end-of-life decision making even if all legal formalities are not met. A living will or surrogate should not be consulted if the patient retains decision-making capacity unless expressly authorized by the patient. Oral statements previously made by the patient can also be legally valid advance directives. |
| • If a physician prescribes or administers high doses of medication to relieve pain or other discomfort in a terminally ill patient, resulting in death, he/she will be criminally prosecuted. | • If a patient inadvertently dies from the use of high doses of medication intended to treat pain, the physician has not committed murder or physician-assisted suicide. |
| • When a terminally ill patient's suffering is overwhelming despite palliative care, and he/she requests a hastened death, there are no legally permissible options to end suffering | • Although physician-assisted suicide is illegal in most states, sedation to relieve suffering is a legal option to treat otherwise intractable symptoms in the imminently dying. |
| • The 1997 Supreme Court decision outlawed physician-assisted suicide. | • Physician-assisted suicide is currently legal in Oregon. Other states are free to legalize or prohibit it. |

Meisel A, Snyder L, Quill T. Seven legal barriers to end-of-life care: myths, realities and grains of truth. *JAMA*. 2000; 284 (19): 2495–2501. For the American College of Physicians-American Society of Internal Medicine End-of-Life Care Consensus Pane. Copyrighted 2000, American Medical Association. Modified and reprinted with permission.

## Table 86. Status of Previously Identified Legal Myths (Prevalent in 1991)[118]

| Myth | Current Status |
|---|---|
| • There must be a law authorizing the termination of life support. | • Currently existing law in all 50 states supports the termination of life support for both competent patients and those who have lost decision-making capacity, as long as consensus exists among those who care about the patient that it would be the patient's wish or in his/her best interests. |
| • Termination of life support is murder, assisted suicide, or suicide. | • Termination of life supports is considered to be freeing the patient from unwanted bodily invasion. Death is legally considered to be a result of the patient's underlying disease. The law clearly distinguishes such acts from suicide, physician-assisted suicide, or euthanasia. |
| • A patient must be terminally ill for life support to be stopped. | • The law allows any patient to refuse and treatment that he/she does not want, in the interest of protecting bodily integrity, even if that treatment would be life-sustaining and the patient is not terminally ill. |
| • It is permissible to terminate extraordinary treatments, but not ordinary ones. | • The distinction between ordinary and extraordinary treatments is not relevant as a matter of law or ethics. The patient has a right to terminate any treatment, potentially life-sustaining or not. |
| • It is permissible to withhold treatment, but once started, it must be continued. | • Although many clinicians think and feel differently about these types of actions, the law and medical ethics treat the withholding and the cessation of life-sustaining treatment the same. |
| • Stopping artificial nutrition and hydrations is legally different from stopping other treatments. | • In most states, artificial hydration and nutrition are considered medical treatments, like any other. |
| • Termination of life support requires going to court. | • The courts generally want clinicians to make these decisions without going to court, providing there is a consensus among those who care about the patient about how to proceed. |
| • Living wills are not legal. | • Living will have legal support in all 50 states either through legislation or case law. |

Meisel A, Snyder L, Quill T. Seven legal barriers to end-of-life care: myths, realities and grains of truth. *JAMA*. 2000; 284 (19): 2495–2501. For the American College of Physicians-American Society of Internal Medicine End-of-Life Care Consensus Pane. Copyrighted 2000, American Medical Association. Modified and reprinted with permission.

## Table 87. Advance Directives: Instructive and Proxy

### Instructive Directives

An instructive directive is written by a person with decision-making capacity and becomes effective when the person's capacity to make healthcare decisions is compromised. Examples of instructive directives include living wills, Natural Death Act documents, and medical directives. Some states allow family members to execute a Natural Death Act document after the patient loses decision-making capacity.

*Note:* An advance directive is not synonymous with a physician's order. Physicians should honor the intent of a patient's advance directive and, after consultation with the patient/surrogate, family, and involved others, write appropriate orders (e.g., an order not to resuscitate or to withdraw artificial nutrition when it no longer serves the patient's best interests).

### Proxy Directives

Proxy directives authorize a specific person to make healthcare decisions on behalf of a patient, in the event the patient loses decision-making capacity. Common examples include the durable power of attorney for healthcare and designation of a healthcare surrogate.

In the absence of a proxy directive, most states designate the patient's spouse, then adult children, then parents or siblings to act as the patient's surrogate. Neither the patient's physician nor members of the hospice/palliative care team should serve as a patient's surrogate. A proxy is invaluable in the following circumstances:

- A patient wants someone other than a legal spouse to act as the proxy (e.g., a specific family member, a lover).
- Disagreements among family members cannot be resolved.
- Family members are unavailable or nonexistent.

## Table 88. Misconceptions About CPR and DNR Orders

Patients/surrogates or family members may be reluctant to forgo CPR due to the following misconceptions about the procedure and DNR orders:

- CPR
  - is a benign procedure with no potential risks or burdens
  - always restores life and restores it to its previous level.
- DNR orders mean
  - death is imminent, or somehow a DNR order will cause death to become imminent
  - the patient will be ignored, particularly in an acute-care facility
  - "nothing will be done" when the patient begins to die
  - pain and symptom control measures will cease
  - supportive care will end
  - the patient is ready and willing to die.

## Table 89. Making Decisions Regarding Futile Treatment

Decisions about futility should be made in concert with other healthcare workers, the patient/surrogate, and the patient's family members, only after[119,120]

- Clearly articulating treatment goals
- Employing full disclosure and compassionate honesty when exploring a treatment's likely benefits and burdens from the patient's and family's perspective
- Clarifying misconceptions and unrealistic expectations about specific treatments
- Understanding that a universally accepted definition of the term *futility* does not exist
- Examining why a specific treatment might be unwarranted (futile) (e.g., lack of physiological effect, low likelihood of survival for any meaningful period of time, poor quality of resulting life, prolonged suffering).
- Explicitly stating the values that will inform a decision of futility (e.g., short-term survival is, or is not, a goal worth pursuing)
- Refraining from using the concept of futility to justify the allocation of scarce resources
- Participating in a formal, procedural, institutional review, if differences cannot be resolved.

## Table 90. Forgoing Treatment: Data-Gathering Questions for Physicians[121]

**Ask the family**

- What do you understand about what is going on?
- Why have you decided to ___________?
- What are you hoping we can accomplish/achieve?
- What do you think ___________ would want us to accomplish for him/her?
- What else would he/she want us to accomplish?
- Which of these are the most important?
- In what situations, if any, could you imagine ___________ not wanting to continue to live?
- Are your questions getting answered? Do you have concerns about the care ___________ is getting?
- Are there disagreements among family members?

**Ask yourself**

- What do I think are this patient's chances of surviving to discharge/recovering function?
- What have I told the patient/family are his/her chances of surviving to discharge/recovering function?
- How sure am I about his/her prognosis? On what is it based?
- What do I know about what this patient wants (or would have wanted)? How sure am I?

*continued*

## Table 90. Forgoing Treatment: Data-Gathering Questions for Physicians[121] *(continued)*

**Ask yourself** *(continued)*

- Is this patient competent to make his/her own decisions? How do I know? How sure am I? Could it be fluctuating or reversible incompetence?
- Did I/we contribute to a bad outcome in any way (e.g., missed diagnosis, delayed treatment)?
- How do I feel about discussing this patient's death with him/her (his/her family)?
- Who is this patient's "family doctor"? clergy of choice? primary nurse? social worker?
- Do I feel I have enough time to talk to the patient/family about prognosis, options, and goals?
- What words or phrases have I (or others) used that might be contributing to the conflict? (e.g., "stopping treatment," "comfort measures only," "hopeless")
- What aspects of this patient's life do I feel justify withholding or withdrawing treatment?
- Does the family trust us? If not, why not?

**Ask about social/organizational influences**

- Are there financial pressures on the family?
- Are there financial pressures on the hospital?
- Are there financial pressures on the medical team?
- Are families allowed to see what the patient's day is like?
- Are there any concerns about malpractice or legality?
- Are there cultural or religious differences among the patient/family/physician/hospital?

Goold SD, Williams B, Arnold RM. Conflicts regarding decisions to limit treatment: a differential diagnosis. *JAMA.* 2000;283(7):909–914. 

## Table 91. Ethical Considerations Related to Sedation at the End of Life

- Doing everything possible to free adults and children from intractable pain and other symptoms is an ethical imperative.
- Acknowledging the distress of the family and professional caregivers is an ethical duty, particularly when the patient is a child.
- Honoring the patient's appropriate role in making decisions is an essential component of ethical decision making, even when the patient is a child.
- Effective communication and clear, compassionate explanations of the goals of sedation and its effects on the patient are ethical necessities.

## Table 92. The Process of Therapeutic Sedation at the End of Life

- As soon as refractory symptoms occur (or are likely to occur), clinicians should begin preparing the patient and family with compassionate, recurring discussions of treatment options.
- After the physician (in consultation with palliative care experts) has determined that a symptom is refractory, a time-limited trial of sedation should be discussed with the health-care team, the family, and the patient. Discussions with children should be developmentally appropriate. Caregivers and family members should understand the following:
  - The patient cannot be kept both awake and in a relative state of comfort.
  - Sedation at the end of life is the only reasonable means of providing comfort.
  - Such sedation results in loss of consciousness.
- Family members and staff should voice any concerns, which should be addressed fully with compassionate regard.
- If sedation at the end of life is chosen, all involved staff members must understand the principles involved and follow established guidelines.[122–124]
- If cessation of a short trial of sedation (1–3 days) is followed by a complete return of symptoms, sedation should be re-instituted and should probably continue until the patient dies. On occasion, a family may request that sedation be withdrawn so they can interact with the patient, particularly when the patient is a child. They should be reminded gently that sedation was started because the patient could not be kept both conscious and free of significant distress. Re-emphasizing and re-exploring the goals of care with the family can be helpful.
- If the family continues to request the withdrawal of sedation despite repeated explanations and reassurance, a trial of lower doses of medication is warranted, with the understanding that sedation should resume if the patient appears distressed.
- Even in a sedated state, adults and children can live much longer than expected. Because caregivers may become very weary, planning for adequate rest, food, exercise, and talk with a trusted listener are essential to the well-being of both family members and professional caregivers.

## Table 93. Pharmacologic Principles of Sedation at the End of Life

- Review the medication history to determine if the patient has experienced any significant adverse effects (e.g., paradoxical agitation) with lorazepam or other benzodiazepines. Agitation may be dose related, but once it occurs a different medication is preferable.
- The physician should have experience with the sedating drug (e.g., dosing and titration).
- Meperidine (Pethidine, Demerol) should not be used for sedation at the end of life or for relieving chronic pain because of the potential for neurotoxicity from its metabolite, normeperidine.
- Reassess the effects of sedation frequently and watch for breakthrough symptoms and adverse effects.
- When a patient is receiving opioid therapy, sedation may involve increasing the dose of the opioid. However, opioid tolerance compounded by heightened sympathetic stimulation from the symptom may obviate adequate sedation. Escalated opioid doses may exacerbate unwanted side effects, in which case a second agent may be required. Opioid therapy should continue at a dose that effectively relieves symptoms such as pain or dyspnea.
- When rapid titration is required for severe distress in the terminal phase of life, parenteral dosing should be used, if possible. The titrated dose should be based on a proportion of the last dose given. For example, if a dyspneic patient is receiving 10 mg/h of morphine and is experiencing some relief but is still breathless, a bolus of 15–20 mg (150%–200% of the hourly dose) is reasonable, after which the hourly infusion dose should be increased by approximately 50% to 15 mg/h. If reasonable relief through sedation is not achieved when the medication's maximal effect has occurred (15–30 minutes after IV/SC dosing; 60–90 minutes after enteral immediate-release dosing), the baseline dose and the rescue dose for breakthrough dyspnea can both be doubled. Continue to titrate both the baseline and rescue doses by 50%–200% increments to desired level of sedation or symptom relief.[123]
- When opioids do not result in adequate sedation, simply increasing the dose is unlikely to relieve a symptom or provide enough sedation to achieve relief without accompanying toxicity. Begin a rapidly acting adjuvant agent, such as a neuroleptic (chlorpromazine), benzodiazepine (midazolam, lorazepam or diazepam), or barbiturate (phenobarbital). When the patient has no history of adverse effects with a class of drugs, the selection of a sedating agent is based on route availability, sedating properties, and duration of action.
- When sedation is difficult to achieve, helpful medications include midazolam, thiopental, and propofol. Each has a relatively short time of onset and requires continuous infusion.

# 7. The Hospice/Palliative Medicine Approach to Caring for Patients with HIV/AIDS

## Prognosis

**Table 94**, page 146, lists comorbid illnesses that predict poor outcome in people with HIV disease.

## Treating Opportunistic Infections

See **Table 95**, page 146, for prophylaxis recommendations for opportunistic infections.

## Antiretroviral Therapy

**Table 96**, pages 147-148, lists antiretroviral medications and their side effects.

## Symptom Management

**Table 97**, page 149 lists medications for treating oropharyngeal and esophageal disease in HIV patients. Also, see Table 61, page 110.

## Occupational Exposure to HIV

See **Table 98**, page 150, for recommendations for post-exposure evaluation and treatment following occupational exposure to HIV.

## Table 94. Comorbid Illnesses Predicting Poor Outcome in People with HIV Disease [125–128]

- Cirrhotic decompensation (often related to hepatitis C)
- Non-Hodgkin's lymphoma, if unresponsive to therapy
- Hodgkin's lymphoma, if unresponsive to therapy
- Progressive multifocal leukoencephalopathy
- Primary central nervous system lymphoma
- Any metastatic neoplasm
- Intractable substance abuse
- Any opportunistic infection unresponsive to therapy

## Table 95. Prophylaxis Recommendations for Opportunistic Infections [129,130]

| Organism | Medication | Dosage | CD4* | Miscellaneous |
|---|---|---|---|---|
| *Cytomegalovirus* | Ganciclovir | 1,000 mg tid | 75–100 | Causes neutropenia. |
| *Mycobacterium avium complex* | Azithromycin or Clarithromycin | 1,200 mg/wk, 500 mg bid | 100 | — |
| *Pneumocystis carinii* | Trimethoprim-Sulfa (TMS), Dapsone, Atovaquone | 1 DS daily or qod, 100 mg qd, 1,500 mg qd | 200 | TMS is superior. TMS allergy may be desensitized. |
| *Toxoplasma gondii* | Trimethorprim-Sulfa | 1 DS daily or qod, or Dapsone 50–100 mg qd and pyrimethamine 50 mg/wk and folinic acid 25 mg/wk | 200 | — |
| *Candidias* | For resistant thrush, consider intravenous amphotericin | 0.5 mg/kg/weekly | — | Premedicate with 500 mg/acetaminophen PO, 50 mg diphenhydramine IV and hydrocortisone (Solu-cortef) 100 mg IV |

*CD4 lymphocyte count below which prophylaxis should be started. For updated information, go to http://www.hopkins-aids.edu

## Table 96. Antiretroviral Medications and Side Effects[131,132]

| Medication | Type of Agent | Usual Dosage | Side Effects |
|---|---|---|---|
| Zidovudine—AZT (Retrovir) | Nucleoside reverse-transcriptase inhibitor (NRTI) | 300 mg bid | Anemia, neutropenia, headache, fatigue, anorexia, lactic acidosis, nausea |
| Didanosine—DDI (Videx) | NRTI | 400 mg qd[1] | Pancreatitis, peripheral neuropathy, nausea, diarrhea, xerostomia |
| Zalcitabine—DDC (Hivid) | NRTI | 0.75 mg tid | Stomatitis, mouth ulcers, pancreatitis, peripheral neuropathy, nausea |
| Stavudine—D4T (Zerit) | NRTI | 20–40 mg bid | Peripheral neuropathy, lactic acidosis |
| Lamivudine—3TC (Epivir) | NRTI | 150 mg bid–300 mg qd[2] | Minimal side effects, nausea, rare central nervous system effects |
| Abacavir—ABC (Ziagen) | NRTI | 300 mg bid | Nausea, hypersensitivity reaction |
| Tenofavir—TDF (Viread) | Nucleotide reverse-transcriptase inhibitor | 300 mg qd | Abdominal pain, diarrhea, nausea, vomiting, flatulence. Rare neuropenia, elevated LFTs, and hyperamylasemia |
| Nevirapine (Viramune) | Non-nucleoside reverse-transcriptase inhibitor (NNRTI) | 200 mg qd x 14 days, then 200 mg bid or 400 mg qd | Rash, hepatitis, nausea |
| Delavirdine (Rescriptor) | NNRTI | 400 mg tid–600 mg bid[3] | Rash, nausea |
| Efavirenz (Sustiva) | NNRTI | 600 mg qhs | Nightmares, nausea, dizziness, rash, central nervous system changes |

*continued*

## Table 96. Antiretroviral Medications and Side Effects[131,132] *(continued)*

| Medication | Type of Agent | Usual Dosage | Side Effects |
|---|---|---|---|
| Saquinavir (Fortovase) | Protease inhibitor (PI) | 1,200 mg bid with high-fat meal or 400– 600 mg with 100–200 mg ritonavir bid[4] | Elevated LFTs, headache, nausea, diarrhea, central nervous system changes |
| Indinavir (Crixivan) | PI | 800 mg q 8 hours on empty stomach or with light meal or 800–1,200 mg with 100-200 ritonavir bid[4] | Nephrolithiasis, abdominal pain, diarrhea, LFTs, headache, dizziness, rash, altered taste, thrombocytopenia, nausea |
| Nelfinavir (Viracept) | PI | 1,250 mg bid | Diarrhea, nausea |
| Amprenavir (Agenerase) | PI | 1,200 mg bid or 600 mg with 100–200 mg ritonavir bid[4] | Nausea, headache, diarrhea |
| Ritonavir (Norvir) | PI | 600 mg bid | Nausea, headache, diarrhea, circumoral paresthesias, elevated LFTs |
| Lopinavir (Kaletra) | PI | 400/100 mg bid | Nausea, diarrhea, rash |

*Notes:*
1. Common dosage
2. Common dosage, not FDA approved
3. Under investigation
4. Ritonavir raises $C_{min}$ of concomitant protease inhibitor, which allows for simplified dosing and may overcome viral resistance.

## Table 97. Medications for Treating Oropharyngeal and Esophageal Disease in HIV Patients

| Condition | Symptom | Medication | Dose | Miscellaneous |
|---|---|---|---|---|
| Oral or esophageal Candidiasis | Altered taste, dysphagia | Fluconazole or Itraconazole | 100–200 mg qd x 7 days | May require doses up to 800 mg/d if resistance develops. |
| Azole-resistant oral or esophageal Candidiasis | Altered taste, dysphagia | Amphotericin B | 0.5 mg/kg weekly | IV administration. Requires pre-medication with acetaminophen 650 mg PO, diphenhydramine 50 mg IM/IV, and hydrocortisone 50 mg IV. Meperidine 25 mg low IV push for shaking chills. |
| Aphthous ulcers | Pain in mouth, odynophagia | Prednisone, Thalidomide | 20 mg qd x 7 days | See Table 61, page 110, for other options |
| Herpetic ulcers | Pain in mouth, odynophagia | Famciclovir or<br>Valacyclovir or<br>Acyclovir | 250 mg tid or<br>500 mg tid or<br>400 mg po 5 x/d | — |
| Cytomegalovirus ulcers | Odynophagia | Prednisone or Fluconazole | 20 mg qd x 7d or 100–200 mg qd x 7 days | Cytomegalovirus frequently colonizes aphthous ulcers or ulcerations caused by candida. Treatment with Ganciclovir is rarely necessary. |

*Note:* See *UNIPAC Seven: The Hospice/Palliative Medicine Approach to Caring for Patients with HIV/AIDS*[7] for more information on caring for patients with HIV/AIDS and the evaluation and treatment of symptoms.

## Table 98. Occupational Exposure to HIV: Recommendations for Post-Exposure Evaluation and Treatment[133]

| Exposure Code (EC) | HIV Status Code (SC) of the Source | Post-Exposure Prophylaxis (PEP) Recommendation |
|---|---|---|
| 1 | 1 | PEP may not be warranted. |
| 1 | 2 | Consider basic regimen; speak with knowledgeable healthcare professional. |
| 2 | 1 | Recommend basic regimen.* |
| 2 | 2 | Recommend expanded regimen. |
| 3 | 1 or 2 | Recommend expanded regimen. |
| Unknown | Unknown | If possible HIV risk + EC 2 or 3, consider basic regimen. |

**Exposure Codes**

- EC 1 = small (exposure of intact skin to blood, bloody fluid, or other potentially infectious material; prolonged exposure of intact skin to large amount of fluid; or exposure of mucous membranes or skin to broken surface with small volume of fluid)
- EC 2 = large (exposure of broken skin to large volume of fluid or other potentially infectious material; or less severe percutaneous exposure (solid-needle or superficial scratch)
- EC 3 = severe (percutaneous exposure to large-bore or hollow needle; deep puncture; visible blood on device; needle previously in the artery or vein of source)

**HIV Status Codes**

- SC 0 = Source is HIV negative.
- SC 1 = Source is HIV positive with low HIV load, on antiretroviral therapy.
- SC 2 = Source has high viral load.
- SC Unknown = HIV status of source is unknown.

**Prophylaxis Regimen**

- Basic Regimen: AZT (300 mg) + lamivudine (150 mg) bid x 4 weeks
- Expanded Regimen: Basic + either nelfinavir 1250 mg po q 12 hours or indinavir 800 mg PO q 8 hours (Due to its half life, indinavir must be given q 8 hours on an empty stomach, not tid.)

**Follow-Up Care**

- Exposed person should practice safe sex or abstain until 6-month post-serology is negative.
- Healthcare workers should receive baseline test followed by repeat serologies at 6 weeks, 3 months, and 6 months (conversion usually occurs 2–6 weeks after exposure).
- Symptoms of conversion include fever, adenopathy, pharyngitis, rash, myalgias/arthralgias, diarrhea, headache, nausea/vomiting, hepatosplenomegaly, and thrush.

*Some HIV clinicians recommend using the expanded regimen for any percutaneous exposure from an HIV-infected source.

*Note:* Up-to-date information is available through the Centers for Disease Control (CDC) Web site at www.cdc.gov/mmwr/preview/mmwrhtml/00052722.htm.

# 8. The Hospice/Palliative Medicine Approach to Caring for Pediatric Patients

## Causes of Death

See **Table 99**, page 152, for causes of childhood death by age in the United States.

## Proposed Continuum of Care

See **Figure 4**, page 153, for a proposed continuum of pediatric palliative care. Although the figure refers to palliative care for infants, children, and adolescents with HIV, the continuum is applicable regardless of the child's illness.

## Communicating with Children

Both the child and the child's parents benefit from clear, compassionate communication and ongoing emotional support during the course of the child's illness. See **Table 100**, page 154, for suggestions for supporting an ill child. **Table 101**, page 155, lists phases in a sick child's acquisition of information and the critical events influencing understanding of the illness. See **Table 102**, pages 156–157, for a well child's concepts of death and supportive interventions.

## Pediatric Pain Assessment and Management

### Assessment of Pain in Pediatric Patients

See **Table 103**, page 158, for misconceptions about assessing and managing pain in the pediatric population.

When assessing pain in children, developmentally approporiate assessment tools must be used. See **Table 104**, pages 159–160, and **Figures 5–7**, page 161 for examples. See *UNIPAC Eight: The Hospice/Palliative Medicine Approach to Caring for Pediatric Patients*[8] for more information and other examples.

### Procedure-Related Pain

For pharmacologic options for managing procedure-related pain, see **Table 105**, page 162.

## Equianalgesic and Starting Doses of Opioids

For information on equianalgesic and strating doses of opioids for children and opioid-naïve adults, see **Chapter 3, Table 41**, page 78.

## Adjuvant Drugs for Treating Pain and Other Symptoms in the Pediatric Population

See **Table 106**, pages 166–171, for adjuvant drugs for the treatment of pain and other symptoms in the pediatric population.

**Table 99. Causes of Childhood Death by Age in the United States, 1998**[134]

| Age Groups | Number of Deaths | Most Frequent Causes |
|---|---|---|
| 0–1 year | 28,488 | Congenital abnormalities, prematurity, labor/delivery-related events, perinatal infections, sudden infant death syndrome |
| 1–14 years | 12,895 | Trauma (accidents, homicides, suicides) neoplasms, congenital abnormalities |
| 15–19 years | 13,627 | Trauma (accidents, homicides, suicides), neoplasms, diseases of the heart |
| **Total** | **55,010** | |

**Figure 4. Continuum of Palliative Care in HIV-Infected Infants, Children, and Adolescents[135]**

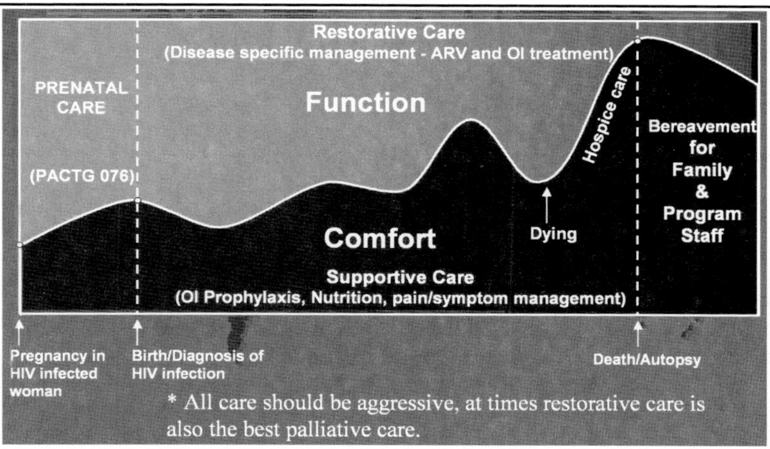


From Oleske JM, Czarniecki L. Continuum of palliative care: lessons from caring for children infected with HIV-1. *Lancet.* 1999;354:1287–1291.Reprinted with permission from Elsevier Science.

### Table 100. Suggestions for Supporting an Ill Child[136]

- Listen to what the child needs and wants.
- Children are capable of being in control of their dying process; support them in whatever ways they need.
- Grief work can be facilitated by encouraging the child to participate in the funeral planning, burial arrangements, and other rituals.
- Children are curious about their illness and its prognosis and about dying; provide opportunities for the child to talk.
- Be comfortable with your own beliefs about death and dying so you can approach a child with openness and honesty.
- Let the child control the conversation and set the pace for questioning.
- Look for cues to what the child really wants to talk about.
- Do not just lecture or give information.
- Be truthful.
- Use simple, concrete language.
- Use pictures and stories for gaining and sharing information.
- Be aware that simply giving children the "facts" can be inadequate because of their different sense of reality; always validate a child's understanding of your answers and explanations.
- Be prepared to accept fears and anxieties in children that may seem irrational from an adult perspective.
- Children often have fears related to separation and pain, such as separation from their mother, painful or traumatic procedures, and the deaths of other children. Anticipate these fears and provide opportunities for the child to voice such fears.

**Table 101. Phases in a Sick Child's Acquisition of Information and the Critical Events Influencing Understanding of Illness**[137]

| Phase | Child's Information | Trigger Event | Child's Self-Concept |
|---|---|---|---|
| First | It's a serious illness (not all know the name of the disease) | Parent being informed of diagnosis (parents often are a primary source of information for children) | "I was previously well but am now seriously ill." For children with chronic disease, "I was in my previous state of health but am now seriously ill." |
| Second | The names of the drugs used in treatment, how they are given, and their side-effects | Parents being informed that child is in remission or worsening; child speaking to other children with similar illnesses | "I am seriously ill and will get better." |
| Third | Purposes of special procedures and additional treatments consequent to the side-effects of therapy, and the relationship between particular symptoms and procedures | The first relapse or exacerbation | "I am always ill and will get better." |
| Fourth | A larger perspective of the disease as an endless series of relapses or exacerbations and periods of improvement | Several further relapses or exacerbations and periods of improvement | "I am always ill and will never get better." |
| Fifth | The disease as a series of relapses or exacerbations and periods of improvement, ending in death | Child learns of the death of an ill peer | "I am dying." |

*Note:* A child's perception may be influenced by peers with serious illness and by the presence of a chronic disease, such as cystic fibrosis or muscular dystrophy. From the time of diagnosis, the child should be kept informed in a developmentally appropriate manner.

From Bluebond-Langner M. The Private Worlds of Dying Children. Princeton, NJ: Princeton University Press, 1978. Reprinted with permission.

## Table 102. A Well Child's Concepts of Death and Supportive Interventions[137, 139–141]

| Life Period | Characteristics | Predominant Concepts of Death | Supportive Interventions |
|---|---|---|---|
| **Infancy**<br>0–2 years | • No conscious thinking<br>• Limited language<br>• No concept of reality<br>• Experience the world through sensory information<br>• Aware of tension, the unfamiliar, and separation | • No concept of death | • Provide maximum physical relief and comfort.<br>• Provide comfort through sensory input (e.g., touch, rocking, etc.).<br>• Provide comfort with familiar people and transitional objects (e.g., toys). |
| **Early Verbal Childhood**<br>2–6 years | • Magical thinking<br>• May play with stuffed animal by repetitively laying it down "dead," then standing it up "alive" | • See death as reversible<br>• Death is not personalized<br>• Do not believe death could happen to them<br>• May equate death with sleep<br>• May believe they can cause death by their thoughts, such as wishing someone would go away | • Minimize the child's separation from parents or provide reliable and consistent substitutes.<br>• Dispel misconceptions about death as a punishment for bad thoughts or actions and the child's being responsible for the death and therefore guilty due to bad thoughts.<br>• Provide concrete information about the state of being dead (e.g., "a dead person no longer breathes or eats"). |

*continued*

**Table 102. A Well Child's Concepts of Death and Supportive Interventions**[137, 139–141] *(continued)*

| Life Period | Characteristics | Predominant Concepts of Death | Supportive Interventions |
|---|---|---|---|
| **Middle Childhood**<br>7–12 years | • At this stage, the child may request graphic details about death, including burial, decomposition, etc.<br>• Early Stage: Understand causality by "external" causes such as accidents<br>• Later Stage: Understand causality by "internal" causes such as illness | • Personalize death<br>• Aware that death is final and irreversible but capricious<br>• Aware that death can happen to them | • Evaluate for fears of abandonment, destruction, or body mutilation.<br>• May benefit from specifics about the illness and treatments and reassurance that treatments are not punishments.<br>• Maintain access to peers.<br>• Foster child's sense of mastery and sense of control. |
| **Adolescence and Adulthood**<br>older than 12 years | • May have a need to speak about unrealized plans (e.g., school, marriage) | • Understands finality and universality of death but may feel distanced from it<br>• Ability to develop natural, physiological, and theological explanations of death | • Allow ventilation of anger.<br>• Provide privacy.<br>• Support reasonable measures for independence.<br>• Maintain access to peers.<br>• Consider peer support groups. |

Frager G. Pediatric palliative care. In: Joishy SK, ed. *Palliative Medicine Secrets.* Philadelphia: Haley and Belfus Inc., 1999: 157 Modified with permission from Haley and Belfus Inc.
Wass H. Concepts of death; a developmental perspective. In; Wass H. Corr CA, eds. *Childhood and Death,* Washington DC:
Rando, TA. *Grief, Dying and Death: Clinical Interventions for Caregivers.* Champaign, IL: Research Press, 1984: 385–391

**Table 103. Misconceptions About Assessing and Managing Pain in the Pediatric Population**

- Children either do not feel pain in the same way as adults, or they remember it differently.
- A valid assessment of pain and other symptoms in children is not usually possible.
- The risks of respiratory depression and other opioid-induced side effects are generally more profound in children than adults.
- The risks of causing addiction outweigh the benefits of using opioids in children.
- Pain in pediatric patients cannot be managed effectively due to lack of effective medications.

## Table 104. DEGRR® Scale[142,143*]

This scale consists of 15 items in 3 categories or dimensions of behaviors: 9 items specific to pain; 5 related to psychomotor inertia; and 4 related to anxiety. Each item is scored from 0–4, with a total possible score of 60. A score greater than 12 indicates pain.

**Scoring for each item:**

0 The child moves without any difficulty. His movements are supple and easy.

1 The child moves with some difficulty, and sometimes a little unnaturally.

2 The child is careful when making certain movements.

3 The child clearly avoids certain movements and moves, in general, with great care.

4 The child must be helped to avoid unduly painful movements.

**Behaviours Specific to Pain: 6 ITEMS**
**ITEM 1: Unnatural postures**

The child avoids certain painful positions or adopts a particular position in order to relieve a painful area. This item should be studied when the child is sitting or lying down with no physical activity. It should not be confused with the antalgic position during movement.

**ITEM 2: Protection of painful areas**

The child seems continuously to avoid all contact with painful areas.

**ITEM 3: Expressing pain**

This item concerns the way in which the child says he is in pain, either spontaneously or when asked, during the period of observation.

**ITEM 4: Indicating painful areas**

The child locates his pain, either spontaneously or when asked.

**ITEM 5: Pain avoidance when moving**

The child spontaneously avoids all movement or tries not to move part of his body. To be scored during sequences of movements (e.g., walking), possibly induced. Motor slowing should not be noted here.

**ITEM 6: Reactions to examination of the painful area**

When a painful area is examined, the child resists, pulls away, or reacts emotionally. Only the child's reactions to the examination should be noted and not any previous reactions.

**Psychomotor Inertia: 5 ITEMS**
**ITEM 7: Resignation**

The child is resigned to everything that happens to him. He does not try to protest or resist. Should be scored during an unpleasant situation, such as venipuncture.

*continued*

## Table 104. DEGRR® Scale [142,143*] *(continued)*

**ITEM 8: Withdrawal**

The child sometimes 'withdraws into his shell.'

**ITEM 9: Lack of expression**

Concerns the ability of the child to register and express feelings by his tone of voice, eyes, and facial expression. Should be scored when the child is active (e.g., during games, meals and chatter).

**ITEM 10: Lack of interest in surroundings**

Concerns the child's available energy for interaction with his environment.

**ITEM 11: Slowness and paucity of movement**

The child's movements are slow, restricted and rather stiff, even some distance away from painful areas. The trunk and large joints are particularly motionless. Should be scored in relation to a normal child's movements.

**Anxiety Behaviours: 4 ITEMS**

**ITEM 12: Tenseness**

Concerns the degree of nervous tension in the child's body.

**ITEM 13: Hostility****

Measures the child's hostility toward those around him.

**ITEM 14: Wariness at being moved**

When the child is moved for a meal, bath, etc., he is wary, says or shows how he wants to be moved, resists or holds onto the adult's hand.

**ITEM 15: Crying easily**

Concerns the extent to which the child cries in order to express himself.

**Comments:**

---

* This scale also can be used to assess pain in adult patients with dementia or delirium.

* * *Irritability* may be a more appropriate descriptive word for this behavior.

From Gauvain-Piquard A, Rodary C, Rezvani A, Serbouti S. The development of the DEGRR: A scale to assess pain in young children. *European J Pain.* 1999;3(2):165–176. Reprinted by permission of the publisher, WB Saunders.

## Figure 5. Bieri Faces Scale (0-6)[144]

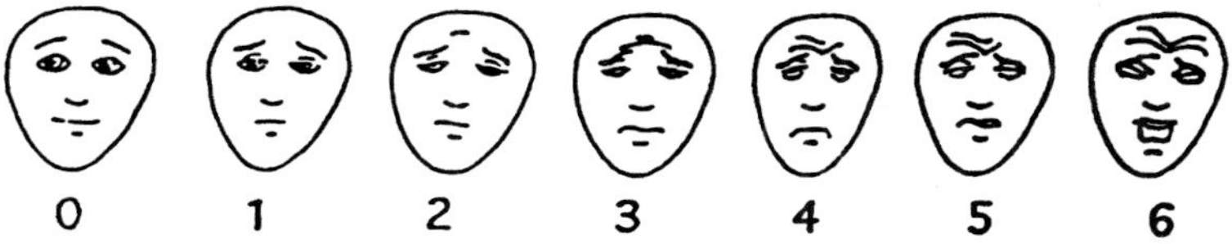


From Bieri D, Reeve RA, Champion GD, et al. The Faces Pain Scale for the self-assessment of the severity of pain experienced by children: Development, initial validation, and preliminary investigation for ratio scale properties. *Pain.* 1990;41:139–150. Reprinted with permission from Elsevier Science.

## Figure 6. Visual Analog Scale (VAS)

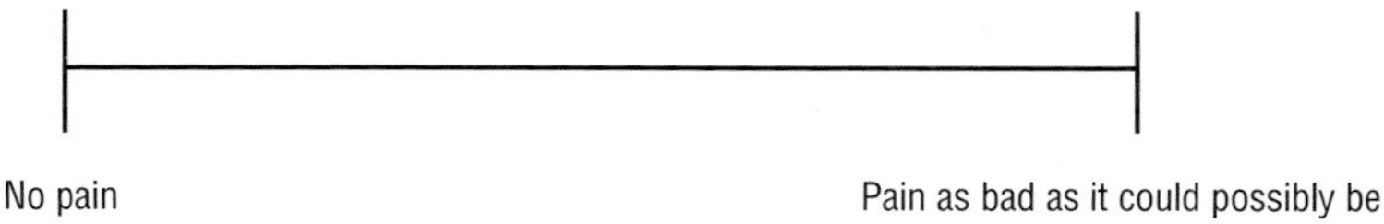


## Figure 7. Numeric Pain Intensity Scale (0–10)

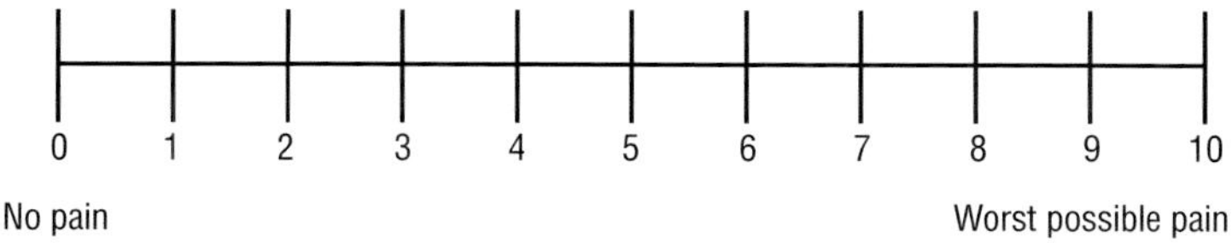

**Table 105. Pharmacologic Options for Procedure-Related Pain and Anxiety***

| Medication by Class | PO Dose | Timing before Procedure | IV/SC Dose |
|---|---|---|---|
| **Class: Benzodiazepine:** Sedative hypnotics should not be used by themselves for a painful anesthetics. | | | |
| Diazepam | 0.2 mg/kg to max of 10 mg | 45–60 minutes | 0.1–0.2 mg/kg peak effect: 2 minutes lasts 2–6 hours |
| Midazolam | 0.3–0.5 mg/kg to max of 15 mg | 30–45 minutes | • 0.05 mg/kg<br>• May repeat x2<br>• Max 0.15 mg/kg |
| **Class: Opioid:** Start with the lower range dose and titrate if first dose ineffective. | | | |
| Morphine | 0.15–0.3 mg/kg | 45–60 minutes | 0.05–0.1 mg/kg |
| Fentanyl | Oral/trans-mucosal: 15 mcg/kg to max of 400 mcg | 20–40 minutes | 0.5–1 mcg/kg IV |
| **Class: Local anesthetics:** Topical and subdermal. These are of benefit even when the patient is receiving | | | |
| Lidocaine & bicarbonate | Not applicable | 10–20 minutes | Dilute 1 pt. bicarbonate to 9 parts of lidocaine<br>Inject subdermally at site of anticipated LP, IV, or bone marrow aspiration |
| EMLA | Applied to intact skin, not rubbed in, with occlusive dressing covering | | Not applicable |

| Timing before Procedure | Comments |
| --- | --- |
| procedure. If the procedure will be painful, use hypnotics in combination with an opioid or local | |
| 1–2 minutes before procedure | • Long-acting, requires long recovery/supervision time.<br>• Diazepam stings IV, use diluted via large vein. |
| 3–5 minutes | • Can use the IV preparation orally by mixing with flavored vehicle (acetaminophen elixir or syrup). An oral preparation of midazolam is now available. |
| 5–10 minutes | – |
| 3–5 minutes | • Oral transmucosal fentanyl citrate—30% incidence of facial itching, reversible with antihistamine. 20% incidence of nausea/vomiting.<br>• IV: **Use with care**, administer bolus over 3–5 minutes. Rapid IV or high doses in the opioid naive can cause chest wall rigidity. This is reversible with naloxone, but is a dangerous complication. |
| systemic analgesia as post-procedure pain is reduced. (i.e., at site of bone marrow or lumbar puncture) | |
| | • Buffered lidocaine stings less than plain lidocaine. |
| 1–4 hours before procedure—increased duration needed with increased skin pigmentation | • Vasoconstriction can impede attempts at venous access. Risk of methemoglobinemia, particularly when concurrent with certain medications. Reversible with methylene blue. |

*continued*

## Table 105. Pharmacologic Options for Procedure-Related Pain and Anxiety* *(continued*

| Medication by Class | PO Dose | Timing before Procedure | IV/SC Dose |
|---|---|---|---|
| **Class: Local anesthetics:** Topical and subdermal. These are of benefit even when the patient is receiving | | | |
| Ametop Gel 9% Tetracaine[146] | Occlusive dressing not required (not yet available in U.S.) | | Not Applicable |
| "NUMBY Stuff" Lidocaine 1:100,000 via iontophoresis[147] | Not Applicable | | To depth of 10 mm |

*PO, orally; IV, intravenously; SC, subcutaneously; LP, lumbar puncture.

| Timing before Procedure | Comments |
|---|---|
| systemic analgesia as post-procedure pain is reduced. (i.e., at site of bone marrow or lumbar puncture) | |
| 30 minutes before procedure | • Lasts approximately 4–6 hours. Shorter application time produces vasodilation, lower cost compared with EMLA. |
| 10 minutes before procedure | • Lasts approximately 1+ hours. Requires grounding. Use with care, especially if allergic to sodium metabisulfite |

## Table 106. Adjuvant Drugs for Treating Pain and Other Symptoms in the Pediatric Population[139*]

| Class of Drug | Route | Dosage |
|---|---|---|
| **Psychostimulants** | | |
| Methylphenidate (Ritalin) or Dextroamphetamine | PO | Usual initial dose of 2.5–5 mg q 4 hr<br>Usual maximum dose of 20 mg<br>↑ gently as tolerated by 0.05–0.1 mg/kg per dose |
| **Tricyclic Antidepressants** (If these fail at maximum dose or toxicity occurs, other antidepressants may be tried.) | | |
| Amitriptyline (Elavil) | PO | Usual starting dose of 10 mg qd to tid for 2–3 days, then ↑ by 0.2–0.4 mg/kg to usual maximum of 5 mg/kg/day (or 300 mg/d) |
| Desipramine (Norpramin) | PO | Same as above |
| Nortriptyline (Pamelor) | PO | Usual starting dose 10 mg to usual maximum of 3 mg/kg/day |
| **Anticonvulsants** (These are useful for neuropathic pain, particularly the lancinating kind.) | | |
| Phenytoin (Dilantin) | PO, IV | 5 mg/kg/dose to maximum initial dose of mg ↑ as tolerated to relief<br>"Load" = 15 mg/kg (if PO, divide in 3 doses)<br>Maintenance = 5 mg/kg |
| Carbamazepine (Tegretol) | PO | 5 mg/kg/dose to maximum initial dose of 200 mg<br>↑ by 2–5 mg/kg/dose as tolerated to relief |
| Gabapentin (Neurontin) | PO | 5 mg/kg/dose to maximum initial dose of 300 mg<br>↑ by 2–5 mg/kg/day as tolerated to relief |

| Frequency | Comments |
|---|---|
| q am & noon | • Helpful for counteracting opioid-induced sedation.<br>• Helpful for resolving depression in short time frame.<br>• **Use with care:** can exacerbate dysphoria/agitation.<br>• Schedule for time when patient wishes to be awake. |
| q HS | • Useful for neuropathic pain, particularly the dysesthetic kind.<br>• Can enhance sleep.<br>• Monitor blood levels/EKG if appropriate, considering the goals of care and the stage of illness.<br>• Desipramine is less sedating than amitriptyline.<br>• The reduced half-life of cyclic antidepressants in children may require bid dosing.<br>• Avoid carbamazepine as a co-adjuvant if bone marrow suppression is a concern. |
| bid | • Phenytoin is useful in a pain crisis; patient can be rapidly "loaded" IV/PO (maximum = 1 g).<br>• Use cardiac monitor and care with IV load.<br>• Other anticonvulsants may be tried if phenytoin fails at maximum dose or toxicity occurs. |
| bid | • Monitor carefully for sedation, if combining with tricyclic antidepressants.<br>• Bone marrow depressant |
| Start qd<br>↑ to bid, then tid | • Minimal side effects or drug interactions<br>• Costly |

*continued*

## Table 106. Adjuvant Drugs for Treating Pain and Other Symptoms in the Pediatric Population[139]* *(continued)*

| Class of Drug | Route | Dosage |
|---|---|---|
| **Corticosteroid** | | |
| Dexamethasone (Decadron) | PO, IV | "Load" = 1 mg/kg<br>Maintenance varies 0.1+ mg/kg |
| **Local Anesthetics** | | |
| Mexiletine (Mexitil) | PO | 1 mg/kg, then 1 mg/kg q 2–3 days ↑ as tolerated to relief<br>Usual max = 900 mg/day |
| **Benzodiazepines** | | |
| Clonazepam (Klonopin) | PO | 0.01 mg/kg/dose<br>Usual initial maximum = 0.5 mg/dose, then titrate as needed |
| Lorazepam (Ativan) | IV, PR, PO, SL | 0.02–0.05 mg/kg/dose |
| Diazepam (Valium) | IV, PO, PR | 0.5 mg/kg/dose |
| **Neuroleptic** | | |
| Haloperidol (Haldol) | PO, IV, SC | 0.01 mg/kg/dose<br>0.02 usual daily maximum = 30 mg |
| **Miscellaneous** | | |
| Baclofen | PO | 5 mg/dose ↑ by 5 mg/dose as tolerated<br>Can also be given as epidural |

| Frequency | Comments |
|---|---|
| bid or qid | • In acute pain crisis, can be "loaded" and then decrease to maintenance dose.<br>• May stimulate appetite, improve mood (also dysphoria).<br>• Timing important due to severe long-term adverse effects. |
| bid | • Monitor blood levels, EKG at higher doses.<br>• Gastrointestinal side effects. |
| q 12 hours | • Clonazepam may be helpful with anxiety. Specifically used for opioid-related myoclonus. |
| q 4–8 hours | • Lorazepam and diazepam may be helpful with musculoskeletal spasm, anxiety, nausea (particularly anticipatory). |
| | • Lorazepam available in U.S. as 0.5, 1, and 2 mg tablets. They are scored, and 1/2 tablet can be given orally or sublingually with dosage approximated on a mg/kg basis. |
| q 4–8 hours | • Diazepam irritating via peripheral IV. Use diluted via large vein. (Where available, use Diazemules preparation in peripheral IV.) |
| up to q 8 hours | • Used to relieve delirium, nausea, and vomiting or to produce sedation.<br>• **Use with care:** can cause dystonia (reversible with diphenhydramine 1 mg/kg). |
| bid | • Can increase dose by 5 mg/dose as tolerated.<br>• Can be helpful in neuropathic pain and spasticity.<br>• Can cause sedation; may improve with time.<br>• **Use with care:** abrupt withdrawal symptoms such as hallucinations, seizures, anxiety. |

*continued*

**Table 106. Adjuvant Drugs for Treating Pain and Other Symptoms in the Pediatric Population**[139*] *(continued)*

| Class of Drug | Route | Dosage |
|---|---|---|
| **Biphosphonates** (Because of little pediatric experience with biphosphonate, there are no specific guidelines for children.) | | |
| Pamidronate (Aredia) | IV by infusion | Pediatric dose estimated from usual adult dose of 60–90 mg (approximately 1–2 mg/kg/dose) |
| Alendronate (Fosamax) | PO | Pediatric dose estimated from usual adult dose of 35–70 mg (approximately 0.5mg/kg/dose) weekly or 5–10 mg/daily |
| **Cholinergic Agent** | | |
| Bethanechol (Urecholine) | PO | Initial dose of 2.5–5 mg (up to 10 mg in adults)<br>Repeat hourly until void or maximum of 50 mg or toxicity reached |
| | SC | Initial dose of 1mg (2.5 mg in adults)<br>Repeat Q15–30 min until viod or maximum of 10 mg or toxicity reached. |
| **Topical agents** | | |
| Capsaicin | Topical | Start at 0.025; can increase to 0.075 |
| EMLA | Topical | |

*PO, orally; IV, intravenously; EKG, electrocardiogram; PR, rectally; SL, sublingualy; SC, subcutaneously 1999:157–173. Modified and reprinted with permission from Hanley & Belfus, Inc.

| Frequency | Comments |
|---|---|
| 4 weeks | Dose is extrapolated from adult experience. Primary indication for treatment of hypercalcemia. Patients can be eucalcemic and safely receive treatment. Monitor electrolytes (Ca and $PO_4$). |
| d or q week | Take with plain water only, ½ hour before the first food, drink, or medication of the day. Patients should then stay upright with no food, drink or medication for a further 30+ minutes (Increased risk of esophageal irritation/erosion with supine position.) |
| *Up to 4 times daily | • Used to manage opiod-induced urinary retention.<br>• Preferable to give on an empty stomach as may cause nausea or vomiting *(Cumulative maximum of 50 mg with initial titration, then minimal effective dose can be given 3–4 times/24 hours.) |
| | • More adverse effects with SC route.<br>*Cumulative maximum of 10 mg with initial titration, then minimal effective dose can be given 3–4 times/24 hours. |
| id | • Capsaicin can help alleviate peripheral neuropathic pain.<br>• Capsaicin causes initial discomfort (burning) with application; may be prevented by using EMLA or lidocaine. |
| Usually 1–4 hours | • EMLA (refer to detail in the procedural pain section of *UNIPAC EIGHT*.[8]<br>• May be helpful for neuropathic pain from cutaneous causes (e.g., herpetic neuralgia)<br>• Do not use on skin erosions. |

Frager G. Pediatric palliative care. In: Joishy SK, ed. *Palliative Medicine Secrets*. Philadelphia: Hanley & Belfus;

# References


1. Storey P, Knight CF. *UNIPAC One: The Hospice/Palliative Medicine Approach to End-of-Life Care.* 2nd ed. *Hospice/Palliative Medicine Self-Study Program for Physicians.* Storey P, Knight CF, eds. Larchmont, NY: Mary Ann Liebert; 2003.
2. Storey P, Knight CF. *UNIPAC Two: Alleviating Psychological and Spiritual Pain in the Terminally Ill.* 2nd ed. *Hospice/Palliative Medicine Self-Study Program for Physicians.* Storey P, Knight CF, eds. Larchmont, NY: Mary Ann Liebert; 2003.
3. Storey P, Knight CF. *UNIPAC Three: Assessment and Treatment of Pain in the Terminally Ill.* 2nd ed. *Hospice/Palliative Medicine Self-Study Program for Physicians.* Storey P, Knight CF, eds. Larchmont, NY: Mary Ann Liebert; 2003.
4. Storey P, Knight CF. *UNIPAC Four: Management of Selected Non-pain Symptoms in the Terminally Ill.* 2nd ed. *Hospice/Palliative Medicine Self-Study Program for Physicians.* Storey P, Knight CF, eds. Larchmont, NY: Mary Ann Liebert; 2003.
5. Storey P, Knight CF. *UNIPAC Five: Caring for the Terminally Ill: Communication and the Physician's Role on the Interdisciplinary Team.* 2nd ed. *Hospice/Palliative Medicine Self-Study Program for Physicians.* Storey P, Knight CF, eds. Larchmont, NY: Mary Ann Liebert; 2003.
6. Storey P, Knight CF. *UNIPAC Six: Ethical and Legal Decision Making When Caring for the Terminally Ill.* 2nd ed. *Hospice/Palliative Medicine Self-Study Program for Physicians.* Storey P, Knight CF, eds. Larchmont, NY: Mary Ann Liebert; 2003.
7. Reiter GS, Alexander CS. *UNIPAC Seven: The Hospice/Palliative Medicine Approach to Caring for Patients With HIV/AIDS.* In: *Hospice/Palliative Medicine Self-Study Program for Physicians.* Storey P, Knight CF, eds. Larchmont, NY: Mary Ann Liebert; 2003.
8. Levetown M, Frager G. *UNIPAC Eight. The Hospice/Palliative Medicine Approach to Caring for Pediatric Patients.* In: *Hospice/Palliative Medicine Self-Study Program for Physicians.* Storey P, Knight CF, eds. Larchmont, NY: Mary Ann Liebert; 2003.
9. National Academy of Sciences. *Institute of Medicine. Approaching Death: Improving Care at the End of Life.* Field MJ, Cassel CK, eds. Washington, DC: National Academy Press; 1997.
10. World Health Organization. *Cancer Pain Relief and Palliative Care: Technical Report Series 804.* Geneva: World Health Organization; 1990.
11. Task Force on Palliative Care, Last Acts Campaign Robert Wood Johnson Foundation. Precepts of palliative care. *J Palliat Med.* 1998;1(2):
12. National Hospice Organization. *Standards of a Hospice Program of Care.* Arlington, Va: National Hospice Organization; 1993.

13. Doyle D, Hanks G, MacDonald N. Introduction. In: Doyle D, Hanks G WC, MacDonald N, eds. *Oxford Textbook of Palliative Medicine.* New York: Oxford University Press; 1993:3-8.
14. American Board of Hospice/Palliative Medicine. *Certification Examination in Hospice and Palliative Medicine.* www.abhpm.org
15. Saunders C, ed. *The Management of Terminal Disease.* London: Edward Arnold Ltd; 1978:195-202.
16. Frager G. Pediatric palliative care: building the model, bridging the gaps. *J Palliat Care.* 1996;12 (3): 9-12.
17. *A Guide to the Development of Children's Palliative Care Services.* Report of a joint working party of the Royal College of Paediatrics and Child Health (RCPCH) and Association for Children with Life–Threatening or Terminal Conditions and their Families. London: RCPCH; 1997.
18. *Palliative Care Services.* Report of the Subcommittee on Institutional Program Guidelines. Health Services and Promotion Branch, Health and Welfare Canada; 1989.
19. Downing GM, Braithwaite DL, Wilde JM. Victoria BGY palliative care model—a new model for the 1990's. *J Palliat Care.* 1993;9(4):26-32.
20. Cohen SR, Mount BM, Strobel MG, Bui F. The McGill Quality of Life Questionnaire; a measure of quality of life appropriate for people with advanced disease. A preliminary study of validity and acceptability. *Palliat Med.* 1995;9(3):207-219.
21. Tulsky JA, Steinhauser KE, Bosworth HB, Clipp EC, McNeilly M, Christakis NA. Assessment of a new instrument to measure quality of life at the end of life. *J Palliat Med.* 2002;5(1):206. Abstract.
22. Byock IR. The nature of suffering and the nature of opportunity at the end of life. *Clin Geriatric Med.* 1996;12(2):237-252.
23. Benefits Protection and Improvement Act, subtitle C, section 322, amending section 1814 (a)(7) of the Social Security Act, as quoted in HCFA Program Memorandum to Intermediaries and Carriers, transmittal AB-01-09, 1/24/01.
24. Karnofsky DA, Albelman WH, Craver LP, Burchenal JH. The use of nitrogen mustards in the palliative treatment of carcinoma. *Cancer.* 1948;1:634-656.
25. Reuben DB, Mor V, Hiris J. Clinical symptoms and length of survival in patients with terminal cancer. *Arch Intern Med.* 1988; 148:1586-1591.
26. Oken MM, Creech RH, Tormey DC, Horton J, Davis TE, McFadden ET, Carbone PP. Toxicity and response criteria of The Eastern Cooperative Oncology Group. *Am J Clin Oncol.* 1982;5:649-655.
27. Anderson F, Downing GM, Hill J, Casorsc L, Lerch N. Palliative Performance Scale (PPS): A new tool. *J Palliat Care.* 1996;12(1):5-11.

28. Stuart B, Herbst L, Kinzbrunner B, Predor M, Connor S, Ryndes T. *Medical Guidelines for Determining Prognosis in Selected Non-cancer Diseases,* 2nd ed. National Hospice Organization. 1901 North Moore Street, Suite 901, Arlington, Virginia. 1996.
29. Reisberg B. Functional Assessment Staging Scale (FAST). *Psychopharmacology Bulletin.* 1998;24:653-659.
30. Doyle D. Have we looked beyond the physical and psychosocial? Presented at the International Hospice Institute Seventh Annual Symposium; July 10-14, 1991; Washington, DC.
31. Billings JA, Stoeckle JD. *The Clinical Encounter: A Guide to the Medical Interview and Case Presentation.* Chicago: Year Book Medical Publishers; 1989.
32. Cassell EJ. The nature of suffering and the goals of medicine. *New Engl J Med.* 1982;306(11):639-645.
33. Cassell EJ. The Nature of Suffering and the Goals of Medicine. New York: Oxford University Press; 1991.
34. Kübler-Ross. *On Death and Dying.* New York: Macmillan; 1969.
35. Worden JW. *Grief Counseling and Grief Therapy: A Handbook for the Mental Health Practitioner.* 2nd ed. New York: Springer Publishing; 1991.
36. Parkes CM. Bereavement. In: Doyle D, Hanks GWC, MacDonald N, eds. *Oxford Textbook of Palliative Medicine.* New York: Oxford University Press; 1993:665-678.
37. Showalter SE. Coping with loss. *Am J Hospice Palliat Care.* 1996;13(5);46-48.
38. Lazare A. Unresolved grief. In: Lazare A, ed. *Outpatient Psychiatry: Diagnois and Treatment.* Baltimore; Wilkins and Wilkins; 1979.
39. Dickerson ED, Beneditti C, Davis PM, Grauer PA, Santa-Emma PH, Zafirides P. *Palliative Care Pocket Consultant.* Oxford: Oxford International Centre for Palliative Care; 1999.
40. Bodnar JC, Kiecolt-Glaser J. K. Caregiver depression after bereavement: Chronic stress isn't over when it's over. *Psychology and Aging.* 1994; 9:372-380.
41. Haley WE, LaMonde LA Han, B, Narramore S, Schonwetter, R. Family care-giving in hospice: effects on psychological and health functioning in spousal caregivers for patients with lung cancer or dementia. *Hospice J.* 2001; 15(4) 1–18.
42. Edelstein B, Kalish KD, Drozdick LW, McKee DR. Assessment of depression and bereavement in older adults. In: P.A. Lichtenberg ed. *Handbook of Assessment in Clinical Gerontology.* New York: John Wiley and Sons; 1999:11-58.
43. Callahan C.M, Hendrie H.C, Dittus R.S, Brater D.C, Hui S L. Tierney W.M..Improving treatment of late-life depression in primary care: a randomized clinical trial. *J Am Geriatrics Society.* 1994;42:839-846.

44. Haley W E, West C A C, Wadley V G, Ford G R, White F A, Barrett J J, Harrell L E, Roth D L. Psychological, social, and health impact of caregiving: a comparison of black and white dementia family caregivers and noncaregivers. *Psychology and Aging.* 1995; 10:540-552.
45. Irwin M, Artin KH, Oxmnan MN. Screening for depression in the older adult: criterion validity of the 10-item Center for Epidemiological Studies Depression Scale. *Arch Intern Med.* 1999;159:1701-1704.
46. Lewinsohn PM, Seeley JR, Roberts RE, Allen NB. Center for Epidemiological Studies-Depression Scale (CES-D) as a screening instrument for depression among community-residing older adults. *Psychology and Aging.* 1997;12:277-287.
47. Radloff L S. The CES-D scale: A self report depression scale for research in the general population. *Applied Psychological Measurements.* 1977;1:385-401.
48. Breitbart W, Passik SD. Psychiatric aspects of palliative care. In: Doyle D, Hanks GWC, MacDonald N, eds. *Oxford Textbook of Palliative Medicine.* New York: Oxford University Press; 1993:609-626.
49. Massie MJ, Gagnon P, Holland JC. Depression and suicide in patients with cancer. *J Pain Symptom Manage.* 1994;9(5):325-340.
50. Cherny NI, Coyle N, Foley KM. The treatment of suffering when patients request elective death. *J Palliat Care.* 1994;10(2):71-79.
51. Puchalski CM, Carson DB. Developing curricula in spirituality and medicine. *Academic Med.* 1997;73(9):970-974.
52. Hay MW. Principles in building spiritual assessment tools. *Am J Hospice Palliat Care.* 1989;6(5):25-31.
53. Kellehear A. Spirituality and palliative care: a model of needs. *Palliat Med.* 2000;14:149-155.
54. Hay, MW. Developing Guidelines for Spiritual Caregivers in Hospice: Principles for Spiritual Assessment. Presented at the National Hospice Organization Annual Symposium and Exposition; November 6-9, 1996; Chicago, Ill.
55. Puchalski CM. Spiritual Assessment Tool. *Innovations in End-of-Life Care.* 1999; 1(6):1-2. www2.edu.org/lastacts/assesstool.asp.
56. Meyer, C. *Surviving Death: A Practical Guide to Caring for the Dying & Bereaved.* Mystic, Conn: Twenty-third Publications; 1993.
57. Amenta MO. Spiritual concerns. In: Amenta MO, Bohnet NL, eds. *Nursing Care of the Terminally Ill.* Boston: Little, Brown and Company; 1986:115-161.
58. Kubler-Ross E. Presented at the First International Seminar on Terminal Care; 1976; Montreal. Cited by: Allen, C. Bridging the gulf of meaning: a philosophical approach to palliative care. In: Ajemian I, Mount BM, eds. *Royal Victoria Hospital Manual on Palliative/Hospice Care.* Salem: Ayer; 1982:231-242.
59. Post SG, Puchalski CM, Larson DB. Physicians and patient spirituality: professional boundaries, competency, and ethics. *Ann Intern Med.* 2000; 32(7):578-583.

60. Dagi TF. Prayer, piety, and professional propriety: limits on religious expression in hospitals. *J Clin Ethics.* 1995;6:274-279
61 Puchalski MC. Romer AL. Taking a spiritual history allows clinicians to understand patients more fully. *J Palliat Med.* 2000;3:129-137.
62. Farran CJ, Herth KA, Popovich JM. *Hope and Hopelessness: Critical Clinical Constructs.* Thousand Oaks, Calif: Sage Publications, Inc; 1995.
63. Herth KA. Fostering hope in terminally ill people. *J Advanced Nurs.* 1990;15:1250-1259.
64. Foley KM. Management of cancer pain. In DeVita VT, Hellman S, Rosenberg SA eds. *Cancer: Principles and Practice of Oncology.* 4th ed. Philadelphia: Lippincott, 1993.
65. Pereira J, Bruera E. *The Edmonton Aid to Palliative Care.* Edmonton, Alberta, Canada: Division of Palliative Care, University of Alberta; 1997.
66. Foley KM. Pain assessment and cancer pain syndromes. In: Doyle D, Hanks GW, MacDonald N, eds. *Oxford Textbook of Palliative Medicine.* Oxford Medical Publications. New York. 1993: 148-165.
67. Pain Research Group, Department of Neurology. Madison, Wisconsin; University of Wisconsin-Madison.
68. Jacox A, Carr DB, Payne R, et al. *Management of Cancer Pain: Adults Quick Reference Guide No. 9.* AHCPR Publication No. 94-0593. Rockville, MD. Agency for Health Care Policy and Research, U.S. Department of Health and Human Services. Public Health Service, March 1994:18-19.
69. Kaptchuk TJ. Acupuncture: theory, efficacy, and practice. *Ann Intern Med.* 2002;136:374-383.
70. McCaffery M, Beebe A. *Pain: Clinical Manual for Nursing Practice.* St. Louis: CV Mosby Co.; 1989.
71. Berde C, Ablin A, Glazer J, Miser A, et. al. Report of the Subcommittee on Disease-Related Pain in Childhood Cancer. *Pediatrics.* 1990;86:(5):818-825.
72. Twycross RG. The management of pain in cancer: a guide to drugs and dosages. *Oncology* (Huntingt) 1988;2(4):35-44. Review.
73. Kubisty CA, Arns PA, Wedlund PJ, Branch RA. Pharmacotherapy in liver failure. Chernow B, ed. In: *Critical Care Pharmacotherapy.* Baltimore, Md: Williams and Wilkins; 1995:91-431.
74. Rodighiero V. Effects of liver disease on pharmacokinetics: an update. *Clinical Pharmacokinetics.* 1999:37(5):399-431.
75. Aronoff GR, Berne JS, Brier, ME, Golper, TA, Morrison G, Singer I, Swan SK, Bennett Wm. Drug prescribing in renal failure: dosing guidelines for adults. American College of Physicians–American Society of Internal Medicine, Philadelphia, 2002.
76. Chernow B, ed. Pharmacotherapy in renal failure. In: *Critical Care Pharmacotherapy.* Williams and Wilkins: Baltimore, Md; 1995:45-90.

77. Swan SK, Bennett WM. Use of drugs in patients with renal failure. In: Schrier RW, Gottschalk CW, eds. *Diseases of the Kidney*, 6th ed, Vol III. Little Brown and Company: Boston; 1997:2963-3017.

78. Mathew P, Storey P. Subcutaneous methadone in terminally ill patients: manageable local toxicity. *J Pain Symptom Manage.* 1999;18(1):49-52.

79. Rysamonti C, Zecca E, Bruera E. An update on the clinical use of methadone. *Pain.* 1997,70:109-115.

80. Mathew P, Storey P. Subcutaneous methadone in terminally ill patients: manageable local toxicity. *J Pain Symptom Manage.* 1999;18:49-52.

81. Bruera E. Neumann CM. Role of methadone in the management of pain in cancer patients. *Oncology.* 1999;13(9):1275-82.

82. Bruera E, Neumann CM. Role of methadone in the management of pain in cancer patients. *Oncology.* 1999;13(9):1275-82.

83. Bruera E. Research in symptoms other than pain. In: Doyle D, Hanks GWC, MacDonald N, eds. *Oxford Textbook of Palliative Medicine.* New York: Oxford University Press; 1993:87-92.

84. Portenoy RK, Thaler HT, Kornblith AB, Lepore JM, Friedlander-Klar H, Coyle N, Smart-Curley T, Kemeny N, Norton L, Hoskins W, Scher H. Symptom prevalence, characteristics and distress in a cancer population. *Qual of Life Res.* 1994;3:183-189.

85. Pereira J, Bruera E. *The Edmondton Aid to Palliative Care.* Edmonton, Alberta, Canada: Division of Palliative Care. University of Alberta; 1997.

86. Dickerson ED, Benedetti C, Davis MP, Grauer PA, Santa-Emma PH, Zafirides P. *Palliative Care Pocket Consultant.* Oxford: Oxford International Centre for Palliative Care; 1999.

87. Mercadante S, Spoldi E, Caraceni A, Maddaloni S, Simonetti MT. Ocetreotide in relieving gastrointestinal symptoms due to bowel obstruction. *Palliat Med.* 1993;7:295-299.

88. Kaplan E. A process approach to neuropsychological assessment. In: Bull T, Bryant BK, eds. *Clinical Neuropsychology and Brain Function: Research, Measurement, and Practice.* Washington DC: American Psychological Association;1988:129-167.

89. Freedman M, Leach L, Kaplan E, Winocur G, Shulman KI, Delis DC. *Clock Drawing, A Neuropsychological Analysis.* New York: Oxford University Press; 1994:3-9.

90. Breitbart W, Bruera E, Chochinov H, Lynch M. Neuropsychiatric syndromes and psychological symptoms in patients with advanced cancer. *J Pain Symptom Manage.* 1995;10(2):131-141.

91. Bottomley DM, Hanks GW. Subcutaneous midazolam infusion in palliative care. *J Pain Symptom Manage.* 1990;5:259-261

92. Twycross RG, Lichter I. The terminal phase. In: Doyle D, Hanks GW, MacDonald N, eds. *Oxford Textbook of Palliative Medicine.* New York: Oxford University Press; 1993:651-661.

93. Greene WR, Davis WH. Titrated intravenous barbiturates in the control of symptoms in patients with terminal cancer. *Southern Med J.* 1991;84:332-337.
94. Truog RD, Berde CB, Mitchell C, Grier HE. Barbiturates in the care of the terminally ill. *N Engl J Med.* 1992;327:1678-82.
95. Miller LJ. Oral pilocarpine for radiation-induced xerostomia. *Cancer Bulletin.* 1993;45(6):549-550.
96. Mueller BA, Millheim ET, Farrington EA, Brusko C, Wiser TH. Mucositis management practices for hospitalized patients: national survey results. *J Pain Symptom Manage.* 1995;10(7):510-520.
97. Ellershaw JE, Sutcliffe JM, Saunders CM. Dehydration and the dying patient. *J Pain Symptom Manage.* 1995;10(3):192-197.
98. Fasinger R, MacEachern T, Miller M, Bruera E, Spachynski K, Kuehn N, Hanson J. The use of hypodermoclysis for rehydration in terminally ill cancer patients. *J Pain Symptom Manage.* 1994;9(5):298-302.
99. Gleeson C, Spencer D. Blood transfusion and its benefits in palliative care. *Palliat Med.* 1995;9:307-231.
100. Bruera E, MacEachern T, Ripamonti C, Hanson J. Subcutaneous morphine for dyspnea in cancer patients. *Ann Intern Med.* 1993;119:906-907.
101. Light RW, Muro JR, Sato RI, Stansbury DW, Fischer CE, Brown SE. Effects of oral morphine on breathlessness and exercise tolerance in patients with chronic obstructive pulmonary disease. *Am Rev Respir Dis.* 1989;139:126-133.
102. Portenoy RK, Miaskowski C. Assessment and management of cancer-related fatigue. In: Berger A, Portenoy RK, Weissman DE, eds. Principles and Practice of Supportive Oncology. Philadelphia: Lippincott-Raven Publishers. 1998:109-118.
103. Walker P, Watanabe S, Bruera E. Baclofen, a treatment for chronic hiccup. *J Pain Symptom Manage.* 1998;16:125-132.
104. Johnston M, Earll L, Mitchell E, Morrison V, Wright S. Communicating the diagnosis of motor neurone disease. *Palliat Med.* 1996;10:23-24.
105. Buckman R. Communication in palliative care: a practical guide. In: Doyle D, Hanks GWC, MacDonald N, eds. *Oxford Textbook of Palliative Medicine.* New York: Oxford University Press; 1993:47-61.
106. Ajemian I. The interdisciplinary team. In: Doyle D, Hanks GWC, MacDonald N, eds. *Oxford Textbook of Palliative Medicine.* New York: Oxford University Press; 1993:17-29.
107. Juliá MC, Thompson A. Essential elements of interprofessional teamwork. In: Castro RM, Juliá MC, Platt LJ, Harbaugh GL, Waugaman WR, Thompson A, Jost TS, Bope ET, Williams T, Lee DB, eds. *Interprofessional Care and Collaborative Practice.* Pacific Grove, Calif: Books/Cole Publishing; 1994:43-57.
108. Vachon MLS. Emotional problems in palliative medicine: patient, family, and professional. In: Doyle D, Hanks GWC, MacDonald N, eds. *Oxford Textbook of Palliative Medicine.* New York: Oxford University Press; 1993:577-605.

109. Stedeford A. *Facing Death: Patients, Families and Professionals.* London: William Heineman Medical Books, Ltd.; 1984.

110. White WL. Managing personal and organizational stress in the care of the dying. *Hospice Education Program for Nurses.* U.S. Department of Health and Human Services. DHHS Publication No. HRA 81-27. Adapted from Vachon, MLS. Motivation and stress experienced by staff working with the terminally ill.

111. Quill TE, Williamson PR. Health approaches to physician stress. *Arch Intern Med.* 1990;150:1857-1861.

112. Latimer E. Ethical challenges in cancer care. *J Palliat Care.* 1992;8(1):65-70.

113. The Hastings Center. *Guidelines on the Termination of Life-Sustaining Treatment and the Care of the Dying.* Indiana: Indiana University Press; 1987.

114. MacDonald D. Hospice, entropy, and the 1990s: toward a hospice world view. *Am J Hospice Palliat Care.* 1990; 7(4):39-47.

115. Pellegrino, ED. Toward a virtue-based normative ethics for the health professionals. *Kennedy Institute of Ethics Journal.* 1995;5(3):253-277.

116. Jonsen AR, Siegler M, Winslade WJ. *Clinical Ethics.* New York: Macmillan Publishing co, Inc,; 1982.

117. Scott JF, Lynch J. Bedside assessment of competency in palliative care. *J Palliat Care.* 1994;10(3):101-105.

118. Meisel A, Snyder L, Quill T. Seven legal barriers to end-of-life care: myths, realities and grains of truth. *JAMA.* 2000;284 (19): 2495-2501. For the American College of Physicians-American Society of Internal Medicine End-of-Life Care Consensus Panel.

119. Halevy A, Brody B. A multi-institution collaborative policy on medical futility. *JAMA.* 1996;276(7):571-574. Policy Perspectives.

120. Truog RD, Brett AS, Frader J. *N Engl J Med.* 1992;326(23):1560-1564. Sounding Board.

121. Goold SD, Williams B, Arnold RM. Conflicts regarding decisions to limit treatment: a differential diagnosis. *JAMA.* 2000;283(7):909-914.

122. Cherny NI, Portenoy RK. Sedation in the management of refractory symptoms: guidelines for evaluation and treatment. *J Palliat Care.* 1994;10(2):31-38.

123. Kenny N, Frager G. Refractory symptoms and terminal sedation in children: ethical issues and practical management. *J Palliat Care.* 1996;12:40-45.

124. Siever, B.A. Pain management and potentially life-shortening analgesia in the terminally ill child: the ethical implications for pediatric nurses. *J Pediatr Nurs.* 1994;9(5):307-312.

125. Reiter G, Gardner E, Wojtusik L, Wojnarowski C. HAART Treatment Yields No AIDS Death in an Inner-City Population Over Three Years. Presented at: DART 2000, Frontiers in Drug Development for Antiretroviral Therapy, San Juan, Puerto Rico. December 17-21, 2000. Oral Presentation 045.

126. Justice AC, Chang CC, Becker S, et. Al. Sensitivity of CD4 Cell Count and Viral Load in Predicting Mortality in the Post-HAART Era. Presented at: ICAAC 1999. San Francisco, California. September, 1999. Abstract no. 125.

127. Reiter G, Stewart K, Bangsberg D, et. Al. Elements of success in HIV clinical care– multiple interventions that promote adherence. *Topics HIV Med.* 2000; 8(5):21-30.

128. Stuart B, Herbst L, Kinzbrunner B, Predor M, Connor S, Ryndes T. *Medical Guidelines for Determining Prognosis in Selected Non-cancer Diseases,* 2nd ed. National Hospice Organization. 1901 North Moore Street, Suite 901, Arlington, Virginia. 1996.

129. USPHS/IDS Guidelines for the Prevention of Opportunistic Infection in Persons Infected With Human Immunodeficiency Virus. www.hivatis.org/guidelines/other/ois/oignov27.pdf

130. Centers for Disease Control and Prevention, Health Resources and Services Administration, National Institute on Drug Abuse, Substance Abuse and Mental Health Services Administration. *HIV Prevention Bulletin: Medical Advice for Persons Who Inject Illicit Drugs.* Washington DC: U.S. Department of Health and Human Services Public Health Service, 1997.

131. Bartlett J, Gallant J. *2000-2001 Medical Management of HIV Infection.* Johns Hopkins University. Department of Infectious Diseases. Baltimore, Md; Port City Press: 2001.

132. *Physicians' Desk Reference.* 55th ed. Montvale, NJ; Medical Economics Company, Inc: 2001.

133. Centers for Disease Control and Prevention. Public Health Service guidelines for the management of health-care worker exposure to HIV and recommendations for postexposure prophylaxis. MMWR. 1998;47 (May 15, RR-7):1-28.

134. Guyer B, Hoyert DL, Martin JA, Ventura SJ, MacDormzn MF, Strobino DM. Annual Summary of Vital Statistics – 1998. *Pediatrics.* 1998;103:1229-1246.

135. Oleske JM, Czarniecki L. Continuum of palliative care: lessons from caring for children infected with HIV-1. *Lancet.* 1999;354:1287-1291.

136 Davies B, Steele R. Families in pediatric palliative care. In: Portenoy RK, Bruera E. *Topics in Palliative Care.* New York; University Press:1998;3:45

137. Bluebond-Langner M. *The Private Worlds of Dying Children.* Princeton, NJ: Princeton University Press, 1978.

138. Stevens M. Psychological adaptation of the dying child. In: Doyle D, Hanks GWC, MacDonald M, eds. *Oxford Textbook of Palliative Medicine.* 2nd ed. New York: Oxford University Press; 1998:1045-1055.

139. Frager G. Pediatric palliative care. In: Palliative Medicine Secrets. Joishy SK, ed. Philadelphia: Haley and Belfus Inc., 1999:157-173.

140. Rando TA. *Grief, Dying and Death: Clinical Interventions for Caregivers.* Champaign, IL: Research Press, 1984:385-391.

141. Wass H. Concepts of death: a developmental perspective. In: Wass H, Corr CA, eds. *Childhood and Death.* Washington DC:Hemisphere Publishing; 1984:4,18.

142. Gauvain-Piquard A, Rodary C, Rezvani A, Serbouti S. The development of the DEGRR: a scale to assess pain in young children. *European J Pain.* 1999;3(2):165-176.

143. Piquard-Gauvin A, Rodary C, Rezvani A, Lemerle J. Establishment of a new rating scale for the evaluation of pain in young children (2 to 6 years) with cancer. *Pain.* 1983; Suppl 2:S25.

144. Bieri D, Reeve RA, Champion GD, et al. The Faces Pain Scale for the self-assessment of the severity of pain experienced by children: development, initial validation, and preliminary investigation for ratio scale properties. *Pain.* 1990;41:139-150.

145. Van Kan HJM, Egberts ACG, Rijinvos WPM. 9% tetracaine versus lidocaine-prilocaine for preventing venipuncture-induced pain in children. *Am J Health-Syst Pharm.* 1997:54:388-392.

146. Zempsky WT, Anand KJS, Sullivan KM, et al. Lidocaine iontophoresis for topical anesthesia before intravenous line placement in children. *J Pediatr.* 1998: 132(6):1061-1063.

# Index to Analgesic Drugs

| *Generic Name* | *Trade Name* |
|---|---|
| Pyranocarboxylic Acids | |
| Etodolac | —76 |
| Pyrrolo-pyrrole | |
| Ketorolac | Toradol, 74, 87 |
| Salicylates | |
| Acetylsalicylic acid (aspirin) | Numerous Trade Names, 72, 109 |
| Choline magnesium trisalicylate | Trilisate, 72 |
| Diflunisal | Dolobid, 72 |
| Salsalate | Disalcid, 72 |
| **Non-opioid analgesic/antipyretics** | |
| Para-aminophenol Derivatives | |
| Acetaminophen and combinations | Tylenol, 71, 72, 85, 87, 114, 149, 163 |
| **Opioids** | |
| Hydromorphone | Dilaudid, 72, 79, 80, 90, 103, 114, 115 |
| Oxymorphone | Numorphan, 78 |
| Morphine | Roxanol, MS Contin, Kadian, Avinza, 71, 78, 81, 85, 87, 90, 91, 94, 103, 112, 114, 115, 124, 144, 162 |
| Codeine | —78, 87, 94, 108, 109, 114 |
| Oxycodone | OxyContin, Percocet, Percodan, Roxicodone, Endocet, Roxicet, 78 |
| Meperidine | Demerol, 94 |
| Propoxyphene | Darvon, 85, 87, 114 |
| Hydrocodone | Lortab, Vicodin, Hycodan, Norco, 78, 114 |

# Index

Equianalgesic chart c̄ Fentanyl, Demerol, Codeine
Cr. Cl. formula
Ca formula